# Parkinson's Caregiver: Strategies That Sustain

# Parkinson's Caregiver: Strategies That Sustain

*DONNA HAUGER*

**Paperback ISBN:** 979-8-9935566-1-1
**Hard Cover ISBN:** 979-8-9935566-2-8
**E-Book ISBN:** 979-8-9935566-0-4

# Dedication

***To my loving husband, Daryl—***
*For sharing this journey with me, step by step, with courage, tenderness, and unwavering love. This story is ours.*

***To Brian and Kari—***
*For your insight, generosity, and the wish to share life together. Living above your garage in our accessible apartment has been more than practical—it's been a gift of connection and care.*

***To my dear friend, Trudi—***
*Without you, this journey would neither have been possible nor amazing. Your wisdom, presence, and belief in me lit the way.*

*"The simple act of caring is heroic."*
*—Edward Albert*

***And to every caregiver walking this path—***
*May you find strength in your story and peace in your path.*

# Contents

Part II. The Caregiver's Toolbox: Strategies That Sustain Me

# Preface

I didn't set out to write a book. I set out to survive.

When my husband Daryl was diagnosed with Parkinson's, the ground shifted beneath us. The changes came slowly at first—subtle tremors, quiet frustrations—then gathered speed. In 2016, I began journaling, not to publish, but to make sense of what was happening. Writing became my lifeline.

I researched relentlessly—websites, podcasts, and ebooks—gathering information I never imagined I'd need. I was angry, scared, and often heartbroken. I wished I'd known more, sooner. Maybe Daryl's diagnosis wouldn't have been delayed. Maybe we could've prepared differently. Eventually, though, knowledge became power. I learned that protein and levodopa don't mix. That exercise—triking, walking, moving—isn't just good for the soul, it was medicine. That caregiving isn't logistics—it's love, grit, and constant adaptation.

Most of all, I learned that caregivers must care for themselves. It's not optional. You begin as a spouse helping a loved one. But Parkinson's doesn't stay still. It morphs. And one day, you wake up a full-time caregiver.

This book is for those waking up in that role—for spouses, children, friends, and partners learning to cope and endure. I hope these pages offer not just information, but hope. Parkinson's can't be fixed like a leaky faucet. But there are ways to live with it—and even laugh with it. Daryl's laughter still fills our home, reminding me that joy is still here.

# Introduction

Caregiving is not a role most of us prepare for. It arrives quietly at first, then all at once, reshaping daily rhythms, relationships, and even our sense of self. When my husband, Daryl, was diagnosed with Parkinson's, I found myself learning a new language of resilience—one built from trial and error, faith, and the wisdom of others who had walked this path before me.

This book is not a manual, though you will find practical tools here. It is not only a memoir, though you will walk with me through the stories of our family's journey. It is both: a weaving together of lived experience, strategies that sustain me, and spiritual pauses that invite reflection. My hope is that you will find in these pages not just information, but companionship.

You may choose to read straight through, following the arc of our story. Or you may dip into the toolbox chapters when you need something specific—whether it's a reminder to breathe, a strategy for setting boundaries, or a gentle affirmation to carry you through a hard day. The structure is flexible, because caregiving rarely follows a straight line.

Throughout the book, you'll notice moments of pause—prayers, affirmations, or reflections. These are intentional. They are the breaths between the doing, the spaces where we remember that we are more than our responsibilities. I encourage you to linger in them, to let them be as much a part of your journey as the strategies themselves.

For readers using a printed copy, all web resources mentioned throughout the book are listed in the Resources Appendix at the end.

Above all, this book is an offering. To caregivers who feel unseen, to families navigating change, to anyone who has ever wondered how to keep going when life shifts beneath their feet—I want you to know you are not alone. May these words remind you that even in the hardest seasons, there is still joy, still grace, still a way forward.

As you turn the page to Part I, I invite you to pause. Take a breath. Let the noise settle. This book is not a race to the finish—it's a companion for the long road. Whether you're reading in quiet moments or between appointments and responsibilities, know that each chapter is here to meet you where you are.

Caregiving is not linear. It loops, it doubles back, it surprises. So let this book be flexible too. Skip ahead when you need answers. Return to stories when you need comfort. Revisit prayers when your spirit feels thin. There is no wrong way to move through these pages—only your way.

And if you ever feel alone in this journey, remember: these words were written with you in mind. You are part of a quiet, powerful community of caregivers who show up every day with courage, even when it doesn't feel like enough. You are enough.

# PART I
# THE UNRAVELING— WHEN THE FAMILIAR BEGINS TO SLIP AWAY

*"I have no choice about whether or not I have Parkinson's. I have nothing but choices about how I react to it."*
**—Michael J. Fox**

# Chapter One: The Diagnosis That Wouldn't Come

## When Symptoms Whisper

The year was 2016. A persistent hoarseness had settled into Daryl's voice, subtle at first, but unrelenting. His once-brisk stride had slowed to a shuffle, making it difficult to walk beside him. Even my deliberate baby steps couldn't match his pace—I'd find myself ahead, looking back, wondering when the change had begun.

Then came the first outward sign. A neighbor, washing his car in the driveway, paused as I passed by with the mail. "Is Daryl alright?" he asked. "His walking looks more difficult." I offered a quick explanation—his bum knee, a lingering legacy of football and surgery. But inside, I felt a flicker of unease.

The hoarseness gnawed at me. His siblings urged him to see a physician. Eventually, he relented. His internist found no obvious cause and referred him to an ENT. Still no answers. Just a routine of six-month checkups, each one ending with a shrug.

By November 2020, new symptoms emerged. A tremor in his left hand. Arms held stiffly. His shuffle more pronounced. We encouraged him to bring it up at his January physical. He did. But the appointment offered little clarity. His doctor and a medical student observed the tremor and gait, then dismissed them—age-related, maybe an essential tremor which is not a sign of a severe neurological condition, or perhaps, a side effect of medication. They took him off a drug he'd been on for twenty years, hoping it was the culprit.

But something didn't sit right. I remember sitting in that sterile office, listening to a summary that felt rushed, incomplete, almost dismissive. I wasn't just confused—I was unheard. The door had closed, but not the right one.

We urged him to see a neurologist. Each time, he refused. A defiant glare. A firm "no." He was an obedient soldier, like the sergeant he once was. He trusted his medical team. He kept marching.

As the symptoms grew louder, so did our concern. But concern alone couldn't move Daryl. What followed was a season of resistance—one marked by defiance, silence, and the slow erosion of trust in what we thought was a reliable system.

## Refusal and Resolve

Covid restrictions kept our pediatrician daughter and her family at a distance. But our worries grew. Daryl confided new symptoms—loss of smell, indigestion, constipation, small handwriting, erectile dysfunction, an inability to smile.

In February 2021, after vaccinations, she visited. The moment she saw him—the shuffle, the rigid arms, the tremor, the blank expression—she said, "Dad, you need to see a neurologist. You have Parkinson's."

She offered to make the appointment. He refused. Unfazed, she handed him a sticky note with the clinic's number and instructions: "Tell them your insistent daughter says you need a referral." The note sat on his computer, untouched.

Weeks bled into months. His mood grew defiant. Any suggestion to call was met with a resounding "no." I reached my limit. He was an adult. I let go. The note was tossed into the wastebasket beneath his desk.

Then, one day, he asked, "Where's that note?" "It's in the wastebasket," I said. "You didn't call. You refused help." He retrieved it. The next day, he called the nurse, pleading for a specialist. She contacted his physician, who finally agreed to a referral and authorized our daughter to make the call.

May was the earliest appointment. By then, precious time had slipped away—time when treatment could have begun, when his quality of life might have been preserved. Instead, we watched helplessly as the disease crept forward, unchecked. No recommendations. No roadmap. Just silence.

His eventual call to the nurse felt like a breakthrough. But what came next wasn't relief—it was a reckoning. With every delay, every dismissal, we saw the cracks in the system widen. And I couldn't stay silent.

# America Needs to Do Better

I wasn't just disappointed in the diagnosis. I was disappointed in the system. In how easily our concerns were brushed aside. In how many times we had to retell our story, hoping someone would listen.

Transitions between parts of the system were chaotic, not seamless. Months passed between referrals. Specialists operated in silos. No one seemed responsible for coordinating Daryl's overall care. We were caught in a dizzying array of decentralized sectors—each one with its own gatekeeper, its own delay.

Contrast that with my experience at Mayo. I'd gone for evaluation after an M spike appeared in my bloodwork. The initial diagnosis: multiple myeloma. But after three days of coordinated testing, a team of specialists determined I had MGUS—a precursor, yes, but not cancer. The percentage of abnormal cells didn't qualify. I left with clarity, a plan, and peace of mind.

Three days.

Not three years.

Not three referrals.

Not three dismissals.

That's what coordinated care looks like. That's what America needs more of. We weren't asking for miracles. We were asking for someone to connect the dots. To listen. To lead. To treat the whole person, not just the symptom.

We had nearly lost hope. But then, one appointment changed everything. It wasn't just the diagnosis—it was the care, the clarity, the compassion. And it made us wonder: why did it take so long?

## The Turning Point

Everything changed when Daryl finally saw the neurologist. In one appointment, the fog lifted. The tremor, the shuffle, the rigidity—it all made sense. Parkinson's. The diagnosis we'd feared, but also the one we needed.

And then, everything shifted.

The care was extraordinary. Compassionate. Precise. Coordinated.

It shouldn't take years to reach that kind of care. It shouldn't take a daughter's insistence, a sticky note, and a wastebasket resurrection.

America needs to do better. For Daryl. For all of us.

# Chapter Two: The Day the World Tilted

## Hearing Parkinson's Out Loud

Because of COVID restrictions, only one person could accompany Daryl to his appointment, a lonely restriction for what would be a life-altering day. Our daughter, Cheri, the pediatrician, bravely stepped forward into the neurologist's office, while I listened intently from my homegrown office on a conference call. The soft hum of his voice laced with genuine curiosity. He traced Daryl's history with meticulous care, his pen pausing only to meet our gaze. Every question felt like permission to speak our truth. My shoulders slackened on the other end of the line. Relief unfurled behind my ribs. Finally, a plan—a roadmap drawn by someone who knew this terrain.

As the neurologist assessed Daryl, a somber pattern emerged. There was the subtle shuffle in his walk, a left-hand tremor, and arms that hung stiffly by his side. The lack of expression on his face was particularly striking. Cheri's fears were confirmed—the doctor suspected Parkinson's Disease.

To solidify this preliminary diagnosis, the neurologist prescribed Carbidopa-Levodopa, a medication designed to increase dopamine in the brain and improve movement and coordination. For a month, Daryl would take one tablet three times a day, at 6:30 am, 11:30 am, and 4:30 pm, diligently ensuring it was at least 30 minutes before eating to maximize its absorption.

A month later, the difference was remarkable. When Daryl returned to the neurologist, the shuffling gait was gone, replaced by a smoother stride. A flicker of joy returned to his face as smiles, once rare, now appeared occasionally. The masked expression had softened. The neurologist confirmed the diagnosis, explaining a crucial detail: while Daryl had Parkinson's, he wouldn't die from the disease. It would be a companion on his journey, not an end itself. He would live with Parkinson's. However, with advanced Parkinson's comes an increased risk of complications like falls, difficulty swallowing, choking, coughing up secretions, and infections.

With the diagnosis confirmed, we finally had a name for what we were facing—and a plan to meet it head-on. But naming the disease was only the beginning. The next step was learning how to live with it, how to push back against its quiet erosion. That's when we discovered the power of voice, movement, and connection.

## The Sound of Relief: Think LOUD

The neurologist shared the importance of exercise, recommending that Daryl join the Big and Loud Therapy program. He started with Loud Therapy, a four-week program with four sessions weekly, focusing on speech difficulties. Before, Daryl's voice was barely audible, a whisper lost in the quiet. He wanted to speak clearly, but the words seemed to catch in his throat.

His therapist taught him to regain his voice. He practiced saying "ah" loudly, experimenting with different pitches. Everyday phrases, like "I love you. Let's have chicken for supper," became tools for improving his voice. He also read aloud for five minutes daily. The transformation was remarkable. The hoarseness disappeared, replaced by a confident voice that filled the room. He began participating in conversations again. A sign on his bathroom mirror reminded him to "Think LOUD."

With his voice improved, Daryl began Big Therapy. Sixteen sessions focused on regaining control over his body's movements. He did exaggerated motions, stretching his hands, legs, and rotating his trunk, whether standing or seated. The results were notable: his posture improved, his arm swing returned, and he walked faster. He could get in and out of his chair and dress himself with ease. His balance, strength, and endurance grew.

Now, the therapy continues at home. Daryl uses a training DVD, exaggerating his movements. This effort helps retrain his brain, strengthening the neural pathways and reminding it to move with the same ease he had before Parkinson's. Exercise helps slow the disease's progression, preventing Parkinson's from taking away control and the joy of life.

Transitioning from the intensity of Big and Loud Therapy, the American Parkinson Disease Association (APDA)'s PRESS (Parkinson's Roadmap for Education and Support Services) support group on Zoom offered Daryl and me a welcome sense of community and connection. This impactful 8-week program was specifically tailored for individuals recently diagnosed with PD (within the last five years). Facilitated by a trained healthcare professional, the structured sessions created a safe space for sharing experiences, feelings, and crucial coping strategies. Key topics covered included the initial diagnosis, medication management, the importance of exercise, physical symptoms, daily coping and relationships, daily living tips, caregiver support, and building a healthcare team—providing comprehensive guidance and support for individuals navigating the early stages of their Parkinson's journey.

The nature of Parkinson's differs significantly from many other cerebral disorders. Unlike conditions that emerge abruptly or over a short period, Parkinson's disease unfolds slowly, allowing many to lead full lives, thanks in large part to advancements in medication like Carbidopa-Levodopa. This medicine offers a pathway to a more normal lifespan, a stark contrast to earlier years when the prognosis was far less optimistic.

With the diagnosis behind us and therapy underway, we began to settle into a new rhythm. Parkinson's was no longer a mystery—it was a companion, sometimes quiet, sometimes disruptive, always present. As we adjusted routines and leaned into support, I found myself thinking not just about our path, but about the many paths others were walking too. That's when the image of the migration returned—an echo of movement, persistence, and shared terrain.

# Chapter Three: The Migration

## Charting Our Course Through Parkinson's

The Serengeti sun beat down as my daughter and I stood shoulder to shoulder, watching the Great Migration unfold. We were in Tanzania, East Africa—where vast plains stretch beneath an endless sky, and wildebeest move in waves across ancient terrain. A sea of them rolled across the plain—some charging north in tight herds, others straying toward the acacia shade, a few even circling back to find greener grass. No two moved the same, yet every one pressed onward, pulled by instinct and rhythm.

That image stayed with me. It wasn't just the movement—it was the persistence. The way each creature, despite its pace or path, belonged to something larger. Since Daryl's diagnosis, I've returned to that moment often. Parkinson's feels much the same: a shared journey, but so many unique rhythms.

Last spring, Daryl's tremors flared, stalling his steps for weeks. His stride, once smooth from therapy, grew hesitant again. We adjusted—new balance exercises, revised routines, more rest. Then, like the wildebeest rallying after a detour, he found his footing. His younger brother Jeff, diagnosed later, took a different tack. His first warning was a stiff right side, not quivering fingers. His progress has been slower, but remarkably steady. Their paths diverge, yet they walk the same terrain.

And then there's me. Not diagnosed, but migrating all the same. My role shifts daily—caregiver, advocate, partner, witness. I've learned to read the signs: the subtle fatigue behind Daryl's eyes, the quiet resistance when routines grow too rigid. I've learned when to push, when to pause, and when to simply walk beside him. My own migration is quieter, but no less real, and no less important.

As I reflected on our individual paths—mine, Daryl's, Jeff's—I realized we weren't walking alone. The rhythms we found, the detours we navigated, were echoed in the stories of others. And slowly, the migration widened. It became not just ours, but a shared journey with fellow travelers who understood the terrain.

We are not alone. The PRESS support group, the therapists, the specialists—they are fellow travelers. Each voice in those Zoom squares carries its own cadence of grief, hope, and adaptation. We share tips, tears, and the occasional laugh. We remind each other that while Parkinson's is uninvited, it doesn't get to dictate the entire journey.

The migration continues. Some days feel uphill, others like a gentle descent. There are detours—hospital visits, medication changes, emotional weather. But there is also progress. Daryl's voice, once a whisper, now fills the room. His posture, once stooped, now holds a quiet dignity. And in the spaces between appointments and routines, there is still joy—shared meals, quiet walks, the comfort of a hand held without words.

We may not choose the terrain, but we choose how we walk it. With grace. With grit. With the rhythm of those who came before us and those who walk beside us now. The migration is not a sprint. It's a testament—to endurance, to love, and to the quiet power of pressing forward.

At dusk, the wildebeest slowed. The heat softened, the dust settled, and the herd moved as one—steady, deliberate, unhurried. I imagine us there too: Daryl, Jeff, me, and all the others walking this path. Not racing. Not retreating. Just moving forward, together, across the quiet plain.

In the wide arc of our migration, there were moments that felt still—quiet pauses where the weight of change settled in. Beneath the rhythm of adaptation lay a quieter truth: we were losing pieces of the life we once knew. And while we kept walking, grief sometimes walked beside us.

# Chapter Four: When The World Shrinks

## The Mask Behind His Eyes

Mexico had always been a place of renewal. For years, it had been our escape—a sun-drenched landscape etched with laughter, shared meals, and long walks with friends. But in January 2022, the Grand Bliss in Nuevo Vallarta felt different. The joy was still there, but it was threaded with something quieter, heavier.

Trudi, my confidante of five decades, noticed it first. We were sitting poolside when she leaned in, her voice low but urgent. "Donna," she said, "Daryl looks at you squint-eyed, furrowed eyebrows squeezed together, like he's disapproving." I turned to look. She was right. His gaze, once warm and playful, now seemed stern—his eyebrows drawn tight, his face unreadable.

It wasn't disapproval. It was hypomimia—facial masking—a Parkinson's symptom that robs the face of expression. According to the American Parkinson's Disease Association, this mask doesn't reflect the person's true emotions. Daryl might have been feeling sadness, frustration, even tenderness—but his face couldn't show it. That realization hit me like a wave. The man I loved was still there, but the cues I'd relied on for decades were vanishing.

That moment by the pool was more than a revelation—it was a reckoning. If Daryl's face could no longer reflect his feelings, how many other parts of our life together were quietly shifting? The answer came quickly, and painfully, as the trip unfolded.

## The Last Trip to Mexico

The resort, once a haven, became a battleground. The lack of handicapped accessibility was more than an inconvenience—it was a painful reminder of Daryl's shrinking independence. Ramps were scarce, elevators slow, and the terrain uneven. Each step was a negotiation. Each outing, a calculation.

By the end of the week, Daryl turned to me with a quiet finality. "This is my last trip to Mexico," he said. "I won't fly again." His voice was steady, but I felt the ground shift beneath us. Travel had been our shared rhythm, our way of staying connected to the world and to each other. Now, that door was closing.

Even as the door to travel closed, others remained open. In the quiet spaces between loss and acceptance, friendship offered its own kind of refuge. And the ocean, ever constant, reminded me that grace could still rise with the tide.

# Ocean Breezes and Old Friends

Still, there were moments of grace. Trudi and I walked the beach each morning, our feet sinking into wet sand as the waves receded. The ocean breeze cooled our skin, and the rhythmic roar of the surf offered a kind of calm. We talked about everything—our families, our fears, our hopes. Fifty years of friendship had taught us how to hold space for each other.

In the afternoons, the sun baked the beach until we retreated to the pool, laughing like we used to. For a few hours, the weight lifted. Daryl joined us sometimes, his smile faint but real. These moments reminded me that even in decline, connection could still bloom.

Those moments of lightness didn't erase the reality waiting at home. As winter turned to spring, Parkinson's pressed harder. The rhythm of decline returned, and with it, new challenges that tested our strength and our resolve.

# The Rusty Gears of March

By February, the decline accelerated. Daryl's stiffness worsened. He struggled to rise from bed, to stand from a chair. He stopped biking—first at the Athletic Club, then at home on his Terra Trike. A mild case of COVID left him coughing and fatigued, and his neurologist increased his medication.

March brought new challenges. At night, Daryl shuffled

to the bathroom in slow, deliberate steps—baby steps, like the rusty gears of an old bicycle. He leaned on furniture and walls, his body resisting movement. Every two hours, he repeated the journey. By morning, his stiffness was worse, the medication worn off.

We called the neurologist's office. The nurse relayed messages, consulted, and called back days later. By then, Daryl had improved slightly—thanks to hot tub therapy, Big and Loud exercises, and a return to the recumbent bike. He began to believe that exercise, not medication, was the key.

Just as we found a fragile balance—therapy, movement, hope—another wave hit. This time, it wasn't Parkinson's alone. It was something deeper, more dangerous, and it arrived without warning.

## A Breath Too Long

April brought another blow. Daryl's knees, especially the left, were deteriorating. The orthopedic surgeon diagnosed severe arthritis and administered cortisone shots. They helped—for a while.

In May, while visiting his mother in Fergus Falls, Daryl began coughing severely overnight. The drive home was long, with only two stops. The next morning, we planned to get our second COVID boosters. But Daryl called his physician instead. Bronchitis was suspected. Urgent care was recommended.

By noon, he was at the hospital. His daughter met him

there. The diagnosis: bilateral pulmonary embolism. Blood clots had formed in his leg and traveled to both lungs. Xarelto was prescribed.

When the nurse finally said, "You're free to go," Daryl swung his legs over the bed faster than I'd seen in days. He fumbled with the blanket, reached for his shoes before she finished speaking. I felt warmth rush through my chest. I'd been clenching my hands all morning. We were walking out of that place—together. Each step toward the door felt lighter than the last.

We left the hospital with gratitude, but also with caution. The embolism changed everything. Plans had to be postponed, surgeries delayed. And so we entered a new season—not of action, but of waiting.

## Waiting for May

June brought renewed pain. Another cortisone shot was given, but the surgeon warned it would be the last. A total knee replacement was recommended. Daryl's primary care physician, mindful of embolism, advised waiting until May 2023—to ensure the clots had dissolved.

After months of navigating setbacks—declining mobility, hospital visits, and postponed surgeries—we found ourselves craving something brighter. A chance to reclaim joy, even if only for a moment. That's when the idea of graduation gifts became more than tradition—it became a lifeline.

# Chapter Five: Journeys We Didn't Want to End

## Graduation Gifts and Growing Shadows

Anticipating that Parkinson's might one day make travel impossible, we decided to give each grandchild a high school graduation gift they'd never forget: a family vacation of their choosing. In the past, our trips—ten of us in total—were planned by me or my adult children. But this time, the reins were handed to the next generation.

Claire and William, our twin rays of sunshine, took the task seriously. They poured over cruise brochures, their laughter echoing through the room as they imagined Grandpa Daryl grinning from ear to ear, soaking in the Mediterranean sun. But when we asked if he'd join us, his response cut deep: "I'd be a burden."

That sentence—so simple, so heavy—was a painful reminder of Parkinson's quiet advance. Still, we made the reservations, hoping he'd change his mind. When we discovered his airfare would be free and his cabin discounted by 70%, he reconsidered. The reservations were changed. He was coming.

But even then, the disease lingered in the background. Simple choices became monumental hurdles. "I need a few days to think about it," he'd say, his gaze drifting somewhere far away.

Planning the trip was one thing. Living with the uncertainty was another. Parkinson's didn't just challenge Daryl's body—it clouded his confidence, slowed his decisions, and left me holding the weight of what came next.

# The Weight of Indecision

When Daryl hesitates—something Parkinson's has magnified—I find myself revisiting the same question again and again. I repeat the options, reframe the question, wait for clarity. On the surface, I'm calm. But inside, I feel the slow erosion of energy, the quiet ache of responsibility pressing harder each time.

Does he know how much I carry? Not just the logistics, but the emotional labor of holding space for indecision. I remind myself: it's not his fault. The disease clouds judgment, slows processing. Still, there are moments when I feel invisible, like the gears of our life turn only because I keep pushing them forward.

I love him. I choose patience. But some days, I long for a moment where the answer comes easily—where I'm not the only one steering the ship.

Eventually, the decision was made. The cruise was booked, the plans in motion. But even then, Parkinson's had its say—forcing us to reconsider how we'd move through airports, terminals, and cobbled streets. That's when the wheelchair entered the story.

## The Wheelchair We Didn't Want

William chose a July 2022 NCL seven-day Mediterranean cruise, round trip from Barcelona to Italy, France, and Spain. Daryl agreed to go. I purchased a transport wheelchair, which he initially refused. But his orthopedic surgeon was concerned—his knee could give out. Eventually, Daryl relented.

That wheelchair, once a source of contention, became our lifeline. It whisked us through TSA with surprising ease, earned us accommodating seats on every flight, and even tucked neatly into a closet on some planes. At the cruise terminal, it was a golden ticket—ushering us past a sweltering two-hour wait in the heat.

Just when we thought the hardest part was behind us, another wave of doubt rolled in. Parkinson's doesn't just affect the body—it stirs up fear, unpredictability, and the quiet unraveling of plans made in hope.

## The Night He Said No

Three days before departure, we gathered for a late-night meal. The aroma lingered as dishes were cleared. Daryl sat across from me, his face unreadable. Then, in a voice as flat and stern as a judge delivering a sentence, he said, "I am not going on the trip."

My heart plummeted.

I scrambled: "Are you feeling unwell? Is your knee bothering you?" But the truth emerged—finally, clearly. He was gripped by anxiety. A storm of fears swirled around canceled flights, lost luggage, and the looming threat of illness.

It was the first time he'd named his fears so specifically. After settling down, he decided to go. This trip would be a test—if he could manage it, he'd join us for the next one: Australia and New Zealand, chosen by our oldest granddaughter.

He chose to go. And for a moment, we exhaled. But Parkinson's doesn't wait for permission. It showed up in Corsica, uninvited and unrelenting, reminding us that even joy must be navigated with care.


## Corsica: Fear in the Waves


Our first port was Ajaccio, Corsica. The boat we'd reserved had maintenance issues, so another was sent. Daryl needed help stepping in—my son held one arm, my son-in-law the other, lowering him gently.

But the waters were choppy. They slapped against the hull, tossing the boat like a toy in a giant's hand. Each jolt sent a spray across Daryl's face. His knuckles turned white, breath hitching with every lurch. His eyes locked on the distant coastline, wide with desperation.

It was too much.

After that heart-wrenching experience, Daryl opted out of our private tours in Rome and Naples—Pompeii, Mt. Vesuvius, and Sorrento. Parkinson's had been acting up, making his movements unpredictable and his stamina too fragile for long days of sightseeing.

After Corsica, we adjusted. We chose gentler days, shorter outings, and moments of rest. Florence offered a reprieve—a glimpse of what was still possible. But Parkinson's wasn't done testing us.

## Florence and the Fracture

Florence and Pisa unfolded like a dream. Daryl navigated the day with remarkable ease. He admired Michelangelo's David, breathed in the scent of blooming jasmine, and felt the cool marble underfoot as we ascended the Leaning Tower. These moments etched themselves into his memory—proof that joy was still possible.

Then came Cannes.

Determined to preserve his independence, Daryl chose to step from the cruise ship to the tender without the wheelchair. I watched, heart tight with worry, as he moved toward the gap between the boats.

For a breathless second, I believed he'd make it.

Then the tender lurched.

His confident step betrayed, Daryl's right leg plunged between the vessels. The sound—a wet thud, followed by his sharp cry—ripped through me. Two crewmen hauled him back onto the deck. The wound gaped open, raw and brutal, a flash of red against the blue sea.

Medical staff arrived swiftly. I followed them to the ship's emergency room, my mind racing. Daryl winced as they cleaned the wound. An X-ray ruled out fractures, but the recommendation to follow up at home felt distant, not comforting.

We stayed aboard while Palma's beauty shimmered just beyond reach. I sat beside him, holding his hand, masking disappointment with quiet gratitude. It could have been worse. But beneath the surface, a tide of emotions churned—fear, guilt, and the fragile hope that tomorrow might still hold something gentle.

We returned home changed. The trip had offered joy, yes—but also pain, fear, and a sobering glimpse of what lay ahead. And with that clarity came a decision we never wanted to make.

## Back Home, Letting Go

After talking it through with his care team and feeling the pull of worsening symptoms, Daryl made the difficult decision to cancel his trip to Australia and New Zealand.

The disappointment—his and ours—hung heavy in the

room. We mourned the adventures that might have been, if Parkinson's hadn't reared its head.

But looking back, those vacations became more than graduation presents. They were a testament to our family's resilience—a vibrant tapestry woven with laughter, love, and an unwavering determination to create lasting memories with Daryl, even as Parkinson's cast its shadow.

Coming home from the cruise marked more than the end of a journey—it marked the beginning of a new chapter in our caregiving life. The big decisions—where to go, what to cancel—had been made. But what followed were the quieter disturbances. The ones that crept in slowly, reshaping our days not with drama, but with subtle shifts in mood, movement, and meaning. Parkinson's wasn't just changing our plans. It was changing Daryl.

# When Stream Became a River

As the year evolved, I noticed a shift in Daryl's personality from a quiet, kind, patient, even-tempered personality to stern, negative outbursts.

Driving to the Athletic Club, every time the car eased into the left-hand lane, the easy smile, the casual nod that used to accompany left turns were gone, replaced by a stiffened neck, a tightened jaw and a sharp, "Wrong lane!" His tremor became more pronounced during these agitated outbursts.

One day as I was parking on the grass near a soccer field, he—with tightening jaw and narrowed eyes—hollered, "Watch out! You are going to hit that car." I was irritated inside, ready to fume over, as the car was four feet away. Parkinson's was again rearing its head.

When our granddaughter was mowing the lawn with our electric lawn mower for the first time, Daryl, usually so laid-back about yard work, watched with an intensity bordering on obsession, his voice snapping with criticism over every missed blade of grass. It was as if a once placid stream had been replaced by a churning river.

Another outburst occurred during an evening meal of lasagna with our daughter and her family. As we proceeded through the buffet line on the kitchen island, my granddaughter, balancing a plate and trying to spoon lasagna onto it, accidentally dropped a small piece of hamburger on the counter. From across the room, Daryl snapped at Claire, "What's wrong with you? Can't you keep the food on your plate?"

I saw in Claire's tears not just hurt, but confusion—the

kind that comes when someone you love suddenly feels unfamiliar. Claire placed her plate gently by the sink, escaped to the futon in Daryl's office, and sobbed. Refusing to eat with the family, her heart was broken over a small accident that can happen to anyone. No one in her family could console her.

When it was time to go home, I went into the bedroom and explained about Daryl's Parkinson's disease and assured her that she had done nothing wrong. I was sorry that Grandpa had reacted so negatively. I made a plate of dinner for her to eat at home and shared with Daryl how devastated Claire was—that he owed her an apology because what had happened did not warrant such a response. We talked about how Parkinson's was "rearing its head." As Claire entered the kitchen on her way to the car, Daryl apologized.

Beyond the difficulty planning and obvious anger and anxiety shown above, a caregiver may notice other personality changes associated with Parkinson's disease, such as staying focused says the American Parkinson Disease Association. Many become inflexible and overly cautious. It is thought that the lack of dopamine that affects movement also affects changes in personality traits. In support groups I've been in, care partners have witnessed "quick to anger, stubborn, argumentative, verbally abusive, inconsiderate, speaks without thinking about what is being said..."

These emotional shifts weren't isolated. They began to ripple outward—into our routines, our decisions, even our safety. What started as sharp words soon showed up in sharper turns, missed curbs, and moments behind the wheel that made my breath catch. Parkinson's wasn't just changing how Daryl spoke—it was changing how he moved through the world.

## Curbs and Concessions

Talking about being focused—as the weeks went by, the curb seemed to have a magnetic pull on Daryl's car. He'd hit it not once, not twice, but three times. The growing unease solidified into a quiet determination: accompanying him to his ophthalmologist appointment was essential. When suggested, he brushed it off, saying, "I do not need you there." But I stood my ground. "Four ears are better than two for hearing recommendations," I countered, my voice laced with concern. His car crept toward the right lane—curbs now targets, not boundaries. He finally conceded, and I exhaled, a small victory in itself.

The drive to the appointment became a real-time demonstration of anxieties. The freeway was a parking lot, with a major accident up ahead. I focused on the GPS, guiding Daryl through a labyrinth of side streets. His hands, though gripping the wheel, felt stiff, and his gaze seemed fixed straight ahead. A quicker route was found, weaving through the congestion, arriving just in time.

Inside the waiting room, there was a familiar flicker of frustration as Daryl, when asked, insisted his eyes were "fine." I gently interjected, explaining my observations to the doctor, particularly about his peripheral vision to the right. The ophthalmologist performed a series of tests, ultimately revealing not a problem with his eyes themselves, but a slower reaction time and a limited ability to scan left to right—a consequence of Parkinson's affecting his neck mobility. The relief was immense, tinged with the knowledge of a new challenge and a deeper understanding of the hidden battles he'd been fighting on the road.

The battles didn't end with the curbs until after twice playing a dangerous game of chicken with oncoming traffic. The first time was a mistake. The second, almost a disaster. The near-miss—the screech of tires and blare of a horn echoing in the quiet morning—made my breath hitch. It was enough. From then on, without a word, a silent ritual began: Daryl, avoiding my gaze, would simply climb into the rear passenger seat for every journey, the unspoken acknowledgment of his two mistakes hanging between us like a physical weight. Never again has he gotten behind the wheel.

Driving was only one frontier. As Parkinson's crept deeper into Daryl's body, new vulnerabilities emerged—ones harder to talk about, harder to manage, and harder to witness. The road ahead wasn't just external. It was internal, intimate, and often unspoken.

## The Unspoken Battles

But the road wasn't the only terrain becoming treacherous.

Inside his body, Parkinson's carved new paths of vulnerability. The disease tightened its grip on Daryl, the signs becoming impossible to ignore. His world began to shrink. The frequent, unpredictable urge to urinate or the sudden rush of incontinence became a constant worry.

Constipation, a heavy and embarrassing burden, made each day a struggle. Our cherished trike rides, once a source of freedom, were now punctuated by urgent, often desperate stops. Daryl wrestled with the unspoken burden of constipation, his embarrassment a wall between him and his doctors.

It wasn't until our trip to Europe, however, that the dam finally broke. The pain of watching Daryl withdraw from the tours, knowing his shame and fear of sudden fecal incontinence kept him isolated, felt like a constant ache.

Luckily, our daughter, a pediatrician, had packed an osmotic laxative. Using it offered a glimpse of hope. Upon our return, Daryl was encouraged to discuss this with his internal medicine physician, opening a door to further exploration and potential relief.

These physical struggles weren't limited to the body's private systems. They began to show up in the everyday—in the tools Daryl once wielded with ease, in the chores that once gave him pride. Parkinson's was reshaping not just his health, but his sense of self.

# The Weight of the Wrench

The persistent drip of the faucet became more than just an annoyance—it was a quiet heartbreak, a steady reminder of what Daryl could no longer tackle. I watched him stare at it, jaw set, as if sheer will might summon back the strength that used to live in his hands. The wrench, once an extension of his body, now lay untouched on the counter—too heavy, too foreign. I wanted to reach for it, to fix it for him, but part of me hesitated, knowing that doing so might feel like another theft of his independence.

The tangled maze of the dryer hose mocked us from the attic. What used to be a simple chore now loomed like a mountain. I saw the calculation in his eyes—the risk, the dizziness, the fear of falling—and I felt my own chest tighten. I hated that fear had crept into our home, into the spaces where confidence used to live.

Even the light bulb, flickering in the hallway, became a symbol of loss. I steadied the ladder while he climbed, each step a silent prayer. The ladder swayed, and so did my heart. I wanted to call out, to stop him—but I knew what that would cost him. So I held my breath and held the base, hoping my presence could be enough. Each rung he climbed felt like a test—not just of balance, but of identity.

He longed to mow the lawn. I saw it in the way he looked out the window, eyes tracing the uneven grass like a man remembering a dance he could no longer perform. The sun beckoned, but his legs betrayed him, shuffling with reluctant slowness. His feet, once sure and strong, now moved like they were dragging the weight of grief itself.

Daryl, who once took pride in the meticulous upkeep of our home, now watched from the sidelines. I saw the silent struggle behind his eyes—the frustration, the mourning, the quiet recalibration of identity. He had always been the fixer, the one who made things right. Now, those hands trembled with a new uncertainty, and I felt a deep ache—not just for what was lost, but for the courage it took him to keep trying.

As the physical tasks grew heavier, so did the mental ones. The ledger, once a symbol of order and control, now felt like a mountain. And letting go of it wasn't just about paperwork—it was about identity, legacy, and trust.

## Letting Go of the Ledger

In the warm glow of the morning sun playing peek-a-boo through the blinds, Daryl's desk was a chaos of envelopes and half-filled tax forms. His desktop screen sat open, the cursor blinking in restless circles. He leaned in, fingertips skimming the keys as if each letter might vanish. Once a wizard of spreadsheets, he now regarded his mother's taxes and estate paperwork as an impossible mountain to climb. He glanced at me—hope and defeat struggling in his eyes. I held his gaze for a moment, trying to steady the unease rising in my chest. Maybe this was the moment he would finally let someone else carry the load.

"Maybe it's time to ask Philip to take this on," I offered softly.

He exhaled, relief flickering for a moment—then shifted

his attention to a new hurdle. On the screen, a red warning blinked: ACCESS DENIED. I took a slow breath, quietly praying we wouldn't lose our fragile momentum.

Daryl's mother's voice quivered through the phone: "I tried my password three times... now I'm locked out!" Old age had blurred her memory, turning a few clicks into an insurmountable puzzle. Years ago, after her first husband passed, Daryl had gladly shouldered every tax return preparation, trust decision, and frantic phone calls for help. Watching him now, hesitating at each step, I realized how much that strength had cost him over the years. When his youngest brother finally stepped in, a gentle wave of relief washed over me. The burden lifted spoke more eloquently than words ever could.

Even as Daryl released some responsibilities, other changes crept in—quieter, harder to name. His energy waned. His engagement dimmed. And what looked like withdrawal was something deeper: apathy, a symptom that reshaped our family's rhythm in unexpected ways.

## Scentless World

This loss of smell is a common non-motor symptom of Parkinson's Disease and can precede the onset of motor symptoms by years. In Daryl's situation, we did not observe the loss until after diagnosis.

One day, a familiar scent simply... disappeared. It began subtly, a faint whisper fading into silence, until Daryl couldn't detect anything at all. This wasn't just a physical change; it felt like a part of his world, a vibrant layer of experience, had been erased.

The irony was stark: even the alarming scent of an overheating electrical wire from our television—a smell that once would have sent shivers down spines—now meant nothing to him. And the once-comforting aromas, like the warm hug of fresh bread or the tempting sweetness of baking chocolate chip cookies, were now hollow experiences, stripped of their power to delight.

Beyond the everyday losses, a chilling fear began to creep in—the realization that this unseen impairment could have dangerous consequences. The worry that he might not smell the acrid bite of smoke from a hidden fire, the insidious whisper of a gas leak, the dank warning of a plumbing issue, or the silent decay of spoiled food became a constant, unsettling presence in our lives.

With scent gone, taste followed. Meals became muted. Flavors faded. Even the desire to eat began to dissolve, as if the body no longer trusted what the senses could no longer confirm. And what was once a joyful ritual turned into a quiet reckoning—one that left us both hungry, in different ways.

## Hungry in Different Ways

Each evening, when Daryl pushed the plate away, my chest tightened as if someone had wound a steel cable around my heart. I caught the green beans mid-forkful, remembering how he used to close his eyes in delight at their snap and earthiness. Now he glanced up at me with a vacant stare and said, "Something is wrong with these."

A hot knot of grief unspooled behind my ribs. I reached out, fingertips brushing his hand, feeling the tremor there. His appetite—once a source of raucous laughter and shared recipes—had withered to half-portions and silent meals. I swallowed a lump, tasting only worry. Daryl's diminished appetite reflected the impact of his hypogeusia. Foods that were once his favorites now held no appeal, and even familiar flavors turned flat or bitter.

This under-appreciated feature of Parkinson's Disease arises from both shifts in taste perception and a reduced sense of smell. As dopamine levels fall, so does the ability to take pleasure in food—leaving us both hungry, in different ways.

In the quiet moments, when the screen goes dark, the bread loses its warmth, the green beans taste like nothing—I'm learning to listen differently. To find meaning not in what's lost, but in how we respond. In the way we hold hands, even when the flavor is gone.

The losses came quietly—first in conversation, then in scent, then in taste. Each one chipped away at the familiar, leaving behind a version of life that felt thinner, quieter, more fragile. But even as Daryl's world narrowed, mine began to stretch in unexpected ways. I found myself reaching outward—not just for answers, but for connection.

And in that reaching, I discovered something unexpected: a caregiver study that didn't just offer data, but offered me. A place to be seen, heard, and understood. It was the beginning of a new kind of support—one built not on fixing what was broken, but on learning how to live inside the cracks. These quiet losses reshaped our days, but they also reshaped me. In the stillness, I began to reach outward—not just for solutions, but for solidarity. And in that reaching, I found something unexpected: a new kind of support, and a new way to carry the weight.

# Chapter Seven: The Lighthouse in the Fog

## The Breaking Point

It was a sunny morning. Rays of light filtered through the blinds as I sat at my desk, pouring my feelings onto the screen. Suddenly, a tightness gripped my chest—sharp, crushing, relentless. Each breath felt like a knife on the exhale. Within minutes, the pain intensified, as if someone were squeezing and stabbing my heart at once. I froze. Was this a heart attack? A panic attack?

I remembered reading in *Women's Health*: "You'd totally know if you were having a heart attack, right? You'd clutch your left arm in pain, immediately fall down to the floor, and head right to the hospital. Eh, not so much. Heart attacks look way different in women." That article echoed in my mind as I reached for the phone.

My father had suffered four heart attacks before age fifty. I wasn't taking chances. My internist wanted to see me immediately. Blood tests were ordered, including a D-dimer to rule out clotting disorders. A treadmill EKG stress test was scheduled. If the pain worsened, I was to head straight to the ER.

While waiting for the test, I trained like it was an Olympic event—walking daily at the Athletic Club, gradually increasing speed and incline. I told my daughter Cheri, a pediatrician, about my "practice sessions." She was not amused. "Mom, this is not a test you practice for."

On test day, electrodes were placed on my chest, a blood pressure cuff wrapped around my arm. I walked steadily until I reached the target heart rate. I felt strong. Confident. I thought I'd aced it.

The next day, my internist called. "How are you feeling?" she asked. "Great," I replied. "I think I nailed that test." Silence. Then: "The results showed an abnormality. We need to schedule an angiogram."

The procedure involved threading a catheter through an artery, injecting contrast dye, and capturing X-ray images to detect blockages. The results? No coronary artery disease. The stress test had been a false positive.

So what caused the crushing pain? One word: stress.

The study's name flashed on my screen like a neon sign—divine intervention or my own desperate wish? By January 2023, I hadn't recognized myself in weeks. Mornings were spent sketching grocery lists and scheduling medical appointments; afternoons unraveled those plans in the face of Parkinson's unpredictability. My shoulders hunched under the weight of Daryl's cold glare. Frustration pulsed hot through me. "Enough," I muttered to the shadows. Control—my lifeline—had slipped through my fingers like loose sand.

When caregiving began to feel like drowning, I needed something—anything—to break through the fog. That's when the study appeared, not as a solution, but as a lifeline.

# A Flare Sent Into the Dark

Clicking "Apply" was only the beginning. What followed wasn't just information—it was transformation. Slowly, I began to reclaim my breath, my balance, and my awareness.

# Anchored in Awareness

The study unveiled a powerful truth: the ability to anchor in each moment and release the grip of what could not be controlled. My reactions—those were mine to shape. Weekly phone calls and daily links became lifelines, nurturing not just my role as a care partner, but the possibility of a more positive life.

Awareness gave me clarity. But clarity alone wasn't enough. I needed to act—to choose peace, even when chaos knocked at the door.

# The Power to Choose

Instead of reacting instinctively, I learned to respond with deliberate calm. Peace became a choice. Compassion, a practice. Even tough love had its place. Sometimes, choosing not to react at all dissolved the situation's power.

Wisdom began to guide me—clear thought replacing raw emotion.

Choosing peace was a practice. Rewiring my reactions, my beliefs, my patterns—that was the deeper work. And it began with self-awareness.

## Rewiring the Mind

Self-awareness emerged as a quiet strength. I became fiercely determined to dismantle old patterns. Healing demanded repetition. Cultural and familial beliefs were untangled, replaced with new aspirations and a new quality of mind. This was a marathon, not a sprint—each step a stride toward mastery.

As the mental clutter cleared, stillness arrived. Not as silence, but as strength. Meditation became more than a tool—it became a refuge.

## Moments of Stillness, Waves of Change

During meditation, calmness washed over me. Negative thoughts gave way to positive ones, without struggle. I lived more fully in the present—no longer tethered to the past or anxious about the future. Even cravings lost their grip. A single comforting thought could redirect my mind. The transformation deepened with time.

With each breath, each moment of calm, I began to notice something else: progress. Not in leaps, but in small, steady victories.

## Small Victories, Big Shifts

Inspired by the University of California San Diego (UCSD) program, I began to celebrate the small wins: a walk taken, a chapter read, a phone call received. Each one, a triumph. Each one, proof that healing was not only possible—it was already underway.

The study had helped me reclaim my breath, my balance, my voice. But healing the caregiver was only part of the journey. Parkinson's was still with us—reshaping not just our days, but our future. And so, with new clarity and steadier hearts, we turned toward the question we'd been avoiding: Where do we go from here?

# Chapter Eight: A Place to Call Home

## Because Tomorrow Isn't Promised

I can still see that February afternoon—the way the light slanted through the kitchen window, the quiet weight of the moment between us. My hands were folded in my lap, my throat tight. "I love you," I told Daryl, my voice breaking. "And I want us to plan now, so we can enjoy whatever time we have left ... because tomorrow isn't promised."

Tears streaked my cheeks. He nodded slowly, his eyes fixed on mine, Parkinson's quietly shaping the boundaries of our future. We talked of options—where we might live, how we might make the coming years not just bearable, but meaningful.

That conversation opened the door to possibility. We didn't have answers yet, but we had intention. And soon, options began to surface—from coast to heartland.

## California Sun, Midwest Roots

In February 2024, our daughter Cheri found the answer to her dream of retiring early—a lot in San Luis Obispo, a sunny corner of California where she and her husband could move at the end of the school year with their 16-year-old twins. We visited that September, but the journey was brutal for Daryl: the layovers, the cramped seats, the strain in his shoulders as we navigated each airport corridor. No way would a move out of the Midwest work for us.

Meanwhile, in Minneapolis, our son Brian was gently making his case. It would be easier for him to help if we lived nearby. He and Kari scouted houses with mother-in-law suites, but every listing had the same problems: too many stairs, too far from his work.

Then came the ADU idea—a self-contained apartment above the garage. My chest tightened for a beat as I pictured those four-hour round trips fading away. Brian's eyes brightened until they almost sparkled; his grin felt like a beacon slicing through months of worry. "No more long drives when we need backup," he whispered, voice hushed with excitement. I felt a thrill ripple through me, as if sunlight had broken through gray clouds.

Once the decision was made, the reality set in. Moving meant more than packing boxes—it meant letting go of the past, one paper at a time.

## The Weight of Paper and Memory

A contractor sketched out the plan, explaining how prefabricated, insulated wall panels built indoors would shave weeks off construction. The hinge of the garage door clicked in my mind, echoing that sweet promise: help at our doorstep, just steps away from the grandkids. It felt like the right choice—and like the first inhale after holding my breath too long.

The logistics were less romantic. Since Brian's bungalow couldn't expand outward, his garage came down, replaced with a new structure topped by our future home. That meant one thing: downsizing.

Daryl's office was packed with the artifacts of his working life—an L-shaped desk, file drawers, tax returns from decades past, documents from our parents' estates. They were part of his story, and he couldn't bear to "dispose" of them, as he put it.

The afternoon sun slanted through the blinds, catching dust motes as Daryl pawed through a lean tower of envelopes. His fingers quivered, the edges of the bills curled like dead leaves. "Just get rid of everything," he snapped. His voice cracked the hush. My heart slammed against my ribs. Papers tumbled to the floor.

I leaned back against the desk, planted my feet, and pressed my palms flat against my thighs. The world narrowed to breath.

**Inhale:** count one, two, three—my lungs filled, belly rising like a small tide.

**Hold:** four, five—suspending the storm behind my ribs.

**Exhale:** slow as molasses, pushing out the tight coil of panic.

The silence felt different now—calmer, charged with possibility. I rose, scooped up the scattered letters, and offered him a compromise: "Let's sort by date. Keep the tax forms; recycle the rest."

Downsizing was emotional, but temporary living brought its own challenges. We were in transition—between homes, between routines, between versions of ourselves.

## Basement Living and the Long Wait

By August 3, 2024, our four-bedroom home belonged to a new set of grandparents eager to be near their own grandchildren. The ADU wasn't finished yet, so we lived in Brian and Kari's basement—our king bed set up beside the kids' play area. Three months of sharing one bathroom, the sound of small feet overhead, and the constant reminder that our real move was still ahead.

And then, finally, the wait ended. We stepped into our new space—not just a home, but a new rhythm, a new way of being.

## Living Closer to What Matters

November 1st arrived at last. The apartment was ready—fully handicapped accessible, complete with a stair lift for Daryl. As we stepped inside, the space felt both smaller and larger than I'd imagined: compact in square footage, but open to the possibilities of making it ours.

Though the apartment measured just 600 square feet, the soaring ceilings and long, tall windows transformed it into something far grander. Light poured in like a quiet blessing, stretching across the hardwood floors and climbing the walls. The vertical space gave the illusion of breath—room to think, to dream, to simply be. It felt less like a box and more like a sanctuary.

We weren't just moving into a home above the garage. We were stepping into a new version of our life—pared down, closer to family, and tailored to the realities we couldn't change, yet determined to make the most of the time we still held.

The apartment gave us more than proximity—it gave us possibility. With each sunrise filtering through tall windows, I felt the quiet promise of renewal. But settling in wasn't just about unpacking boxes. It was about learning how to live differently—closer to help, closer to family, and closer to the truth of what Parkinson's was asking of both of us. Chapter by chapter, we were rewriting the rhythm of our days.

Settling into our new apartment brought relief, but it didn't pause the progression. Parkinson's followed us through the door, reshaping not just our routines, but our interactions, our emotions, and even the smallest gestures. In this new space, the challenges became quieter—but no less profound. And so, I began to notice the subtle shifts. The tension. The tenderness. The need to name what was happening, so I could learn how to live with it.

# Chapter Nine: Name It to Tame It

## The Turbo Tax Tension

Daryl sat hunched at his desk, eyes fixed on the TurboTax screen. I'd hoped he'd let Brian handle the taxes this year, or maybe hire someone, but the set of his jaw told me he wouldn't. I asked if I could watch—just to learn, in case his Parkinson's made the task harder in the future. He agreed, for a while.

We worked through a few screens together until he misspelled a word. I reminded him how to edit it. His glare was sharp, the air between us snapping tight. My chest clenched. I knew it was time to leave.

Shoes on. Out the door. Around Lake Nokomis, where breezes brushed my skin and goslings waddled after their mothers along the path. The tension in my body loosened with each step. I named what I felt—disappointment, frustration—following the advise of my friend. The words she always quoted— "Name it to tame it," Dr. Siegel's phrase—echoed. My breath slowed. My mind settled into the present: the smell of damp earth, the chorus of birdcalls, the steady rhythm of my feet.

Days later, with Brian's help, the taxes were finally filed—two states this year because of the move. Minnesota refused the electronic filing; Iowa accepted. It was only when estimated taxes were due that Daryl asked for my help again, unable to find the TurboTax file that held the amount. I opened it for him, quietly, and stepped back.

That moment at the lake reminded me how naming my emotions could soften their grip. But while I was learning to tame frustration, Daryl was facing battles of his own—ones that couldn't be walked off. His struggle wasn't with paperwork, but with something far more fundamental: the simple act of swallowing.

# The Choreography of a Bite

Swallowing has become one of Daryl's quiet battles—an invisible struggle that plays out with every bite. His speech-language pathologist has conducted two swallowing studies, each one a strange choreography of barium-laced foods and X-ray video. I sat nearby as he swallowed crackers, pudding, applesauce, and water, watching the screen as the food moved—or didn't—through his throat.

The first test showed trouble with dry foods like crackers; the second revealed difficulty with swallowing a barium pill with water. In both, the food pooled ominously at the back of his throat, lingering too long, threatening to slip where it shouldn't. To solve difficulty taking pills, a thickening powder was prescribed. When added to liquids, it slows the flow rate, allowing the person more time to control the liquid during the swallowing process and preventing it from entering the airway and lungs.

At home, meals have slowed to a careful ritual. Daryl chews deliberately, often pausing with a look of concentration, as if willing his throat to cooperate. After each bite, he takes a sip of water—his prescribed safeguard against aspiration. I watch him sometimes, heart clenched, as he coughs or clears his throat, the sound sharp and unsettling.

Each morning, seated in his favorite recliner, Daryl begins his swallow exercises. "Swallow, squeeze hard with all your might! Push as hard as you can with your tongue against the roof of your mouth while you swallow," his speech-language pathologist has prompted.

The EMST device—a small, unassuming tool—has also become part of his routine. He breathes out forcefully through it, building the strength to protect his lungs from stray bits of food or liquid. The resistance is meant to train his cough reflex, but to me, it feels like a quiet act of defiance—a way of reclaiming control.

He works on tongue exercises, movements that seem simple but carry weight: sticking his tongue out and pulling it back in, sweeping it side to side, swallowing with it gently held between his front teeth. These motions, repeated daily, are meant to strengthen the muscles that once worked without thought. Now, each swallow is an effort, a visualization, a hope that pneumonia won't find its way in.

Watching him do these exercises, I feel a mix of admiration and sorrow. The body that once moved with ease now requires coaxing, training, patience. But Daryl persists. And in that persistence, I see something stronger than muscle—something quietly heroic.

Swallowing was only part of the story. Parkinson's doesn't just complicate meals—it alters the body's quiet rhythms. And sometimes, the smallest signs—like a droplet of saliva—carry the heaviest emotional weight.

# The Napkin Exchange

One day, I noticed the first gleam of moisture on Daryl's chin as he sat in his favorite rocker, sipping his Chocolate Protein Drink. A warm breeze fluttered the blinds, and for a heartbeat, I forgot the slip of saliva pooling at his lip. Then reality pressed in. My heart twisted as I handed him a folded napkin, my own eyes watering with worry and love.

He caught my glance and managed a wry half-smile. "Guess it's part of the package," he murmured. In that moment, our routine napkin exchange felt like a secret handshake—an unspoken promise that we'd face all of Parkinson's strange twists together.

Daryl doesn't drool because he has too much saliva, the speech pathologist explained at Daryl's follow-up appointment, but because Parkinson's slows the automatic movements most of us never think about—including swallowing. Bradykinesia and stiff muscles delay every swallow, so the saliva simply gathers until it overflows. In advanced cases, it can even slip into the lungs and cause pneumonia, which is why she encourages him to keep his swallowing reflex active—chewing gum, sucking on hard candies, sipping water, or even letting an ice cube melt slowly in his mouth.

It's worse when he rests. During naps or in the quiet hours of night, drool slides unnoticed from the corner of his mouth and spreads across the pillow. I started using dark-colored pillowcases on his side of the bed—not for appearance, but so the stains don't surprise him in the morning and so I can treat them before washing. Sometimes I watch the saliva run down his chin and soak the collar of his shirt before he realizes it's there. He keeps handkerchiefs in his pocket but doesn't always reach for them in time. I feel a mix of sadness and protectiveness when I gently wipe his mouth, knowing he would be embarrassed if he were more aware of it.

There are medications that could help, but most come with another unpleasant cost—extreme dry mouth. Daryl already deals with that daily, so for now, we both manage the drooling as best we can, one stained shirt and one dark pillowcase at a time.

Even as we managed the drooling, another challenge emerged—one that touched Daryl's pride and independence. His hands, once steady and skilled, now needed retraining. And with each exercise, he met the tremor not with defeat, but with quiet defiance.

# Dexterity and Defiance

To help manage the tremor in his left hand and make eating and drinking easier, Daryl's occupational therapist, Rachel, introduced a series of hand exercises—small movements with big impact. At first, the routine felt like just another task on an already full plate. But over time, it became something more: a quiet ritual of persistence.

Each morning, Daryl begins by tapping the tip of each finger to his thumb, ten reps, three sets, moving to the other hand, exaggerating the motion like a pianist warming up. It's a way to coax his fingers into working together again.

Then comes the therapy putty—he squeezes it firmly, holds, releases, and repeats, building grip strength with each pulse. Some days, he flattens the putty and buries ten marbles inside, then fishes them out one by one using only his thumb and index finger, placing each marble in a bowl. It's a game of dexterity, training the small muscles needed for writing, buttoning shirts, and picking up the tiniest of objects.

Next, he practices picking up dimes and dropping them into a container—simple, but surprisingly tricky. Finally, he holds a pen in his palm, shifts it to his fingertips, places it to the left, then back to the right, repeating the motion like a slow dance.

When I asked how the exercises were going, he grinned and said with a chuckle, "I get finger exercise playing cards four days a week with my helper, Rahsaan." His laughter—warm and unfiltered—filled the room. And he's right. Playing cards sharpens fine motor skills and hand-eye coordination, but more than that, it brings joy. In the midst of routines and rehab, that joy is its own kind of medicine.

These routines—swallowing exercises, tremor drills, the quiet exchange of napkins—aren't just about managing symptoms. They're about staying present in a life that keeps changing. Each small act, repeated daily, is a kind of vow: to keep showing up, to keep adapting, to keep loving through the awkwardness and the ache. And while Parkinson's continues to redraw the map, we've learned to walk it together—one careful step, one named emotion, one quiet victory at a time.

We had learned to navigate the daily rhythms—swallowing exercises, tremor drills, the quiet exchange of napkins. But even as we found our footing inside the home, another challenge loomed: the revolving door of outside help. Parkinson's didn't just ask us to adapt—it asked us to teach, to advocate, and to find steadiness in the midst of constant change.

# Chapter Ten: Two Hours of Air

## Another New Helper

At 2:00 p.m. sharp, the doorbell rings. I brace myself—another new face. Daryl presses his hand to the button that opens the door, confusion flickering in his eyes. "Another new helper today?" he asks, voice tinged with frustration.

This rotating team was supposed to be our lifeline, but dealing with the revolving door of people and teaching each stranger Daryl's routines was a nightmare. Last week's walker helper, yesterday's foot soaker—always retold for someone new. Consistency slipped through our fingers.

Just when I thought I couldn't explain Daryl's routines one more time, something shifted. A new face arrived—not just with credentials, but with care. And with him came the first glimmer of calm.

## Enter Rahsaan

Then came Rahsaan. He arrived with a soft voice and an iPhone app—a list of Daryl's quirks. He knew to start with his favorite armchair, exactly 15 degrees recline, before slipping his feet into a warm soak. The lemon-scented water lapped at his ankles as he pumiced away the corn on his right heel. Daryl closed his eyes and sighed.

"You see that?" he whispered as he wrapped an ice pack around Daryl's arthritic heel. Daryl nodded, relaxation softening his rigid shoulders. In that instant, I understood the first lesson: prioritize consistency. A familiar face, familiar steps, and the day tip-toed into calm.

Rahsaan's presence didn't just soothe Daryl—it taught me something vital. That consistency isn't a luxury in caregiving—it's a lifeline. And once I saw its power, I knew we had to build on it.

## Consistency, Communication, Education

After we learned that consistency in scheduling made a profound difference in Daryl's day-to-day well-being, I found myself stepping into the role of advocate—not just partner. I began working closely with his care team, gently but persistently, to shape a routine that honored his rhythms and needs. Parkinson's doesn't ask permission to disrupt life, but through collaboration and compassion, we found ways to restore a sense of steadiness. It wasn't just about appointments—it was about dignity, predictability, and peace.

Over the next weeks, I posted his Provider Orders for Life-Sustaining Treatment (POLST) document outlining

Daryl's preferences for no resuscitation and comfort-focused treatment and a one-page routine on the fridge—required routines in green, optional in blue. Any changes? I referred to the updated sheet and realized the second lesson: communicate clearly.

By this time Rahsaan began each visit by asking, "Shall we walk to Bossen Park today or take a neighborhood stroll?" I'd trained every helper on Daryl's subtle Parkinson's signals—when his voice rasps, when his balance shifts. That was the third lesson: educate your caregivers.

Now we have two anchors: Rahsaan four days a week, Joseph on Sundays. They walk Daryl around the block, scrub his feet, ice his heel, play Hearts for two—and give me two guilt-free hours to run errands or circle Lake Nokomis at a brisk pace. When I return, we take a slow trike ride together later, Bosch motor humming beneath us, and I'm not thinking of chores or deadlines—I'm just here, with him.

Respite didn't just give me time—it gave me perspective. In those quiet hours circling Lake Nokomis or pedaling beside Daryl, I began to feel something I hadn't in months: spaciousness. The kind that lets you think, breathe, dream. And in that space, a new question emerged—not just how to care for Daryl, but how to care for myself. Part Two begins there—with the slow, deliberate work of tending to my own heart.

Respite gave me room to breathe, but Parkinson's didn't pause. Even with routines in place and helpers by our side, the map we once relied on—of expectations, habits, and shared understanding—began to blur. And when the map fails, you learn to navigate by instinct, by love, and by the lessons hidden in each detour.

With Rahsaan and Joseph in place, our days found a steadier rhythm. I began to breathe again—two hours at a time, circling Lake Nokomis, reclaiming pieces of myself. But Parkinson's doesn't honor routines. Just when life feels predictable, it redraws the map. And sometimes, even the simplest outing—a trip to Costco, a ride around the lake—can leave us lost in aisles, off course, and searching for a way back.

# Chapter Eleven: When the Map Fails

## Lost in Aisles and Expectations

The day's errands were a whirlwind: dropping donations at Goodwill, returning an item at Walmart, and stocking up at Hy-Vee on sale-priced licorice, hamburger and buns for the delicious pulled pork our son, Brian, had smoked. Costco was the last quick stop. Daryl wanted a hot dog, so two were ordered. Mine was buried under ketchup, onions, and sweet relish.

After finishing the hot dog, I told Daryl, "I'll grab a cart. I only need a few things: tilapia, shrimp, yogurt, and milk. I'll be quick. If you're looking for me, those are the aisles I'll hit before checking out and heading back to the car." No comment was offered. I should have stressed just how quick the stop would be.

Pushing a cart past the checkouts, I spotted Daryl still eating. I decided to swiftly gather the needed items. Reaching the yogurt, I messaged Daryl, "Need blueberries?" No reply. A container of blueberries and some appealing cherries were tossed into the cart. With tilapia, shrimp, yogurt, milk, and fruit now in tow, I tried calling Daryl to say I was checking out. Silence. I checked out, loaded the groceries into cooler bags (it was a sweltering 99 degrees with a 110 heat index), and started the car, blasting the air conditioning. I called Daryl again; a vibration, but no ring. In the backseat pocket, Daryl's fanny pack was spied. His phone was inside. No wonder he hadn't answered.

The car was switched off, and I plunged back into Costco, scanning every row, but Daryl was nowhere. Retreating to the now-cooling car, I decided to wait, hoping he'd eventually find his way. After a tense 20 minutes, Daryl was watched shuffling towards the car in the rearview mirror. He slowly settled into the backseat. The drive home followed. The twenty-minute ride was filled with an unspoken tension. I wondered how long it would be before Daryl acknowledged the ordeal.

Thirty minutes after arriving home, I finally broke the silence. "What happened at Costco?" Daryl responded, "I couldn't find you." We used to have a system: meet where we last saw each other. It failed us spectacularly this time. "What did you learn from this experience?" I asked. Daryl replied "I need a bull ring in my nose." Despite my racing heart, the sweat trickling down my face and chest, and my feeling that might explode, a sweet thought broke through the stress: Daryl still had his sense of humor. I emphasized the importance of carrying his phone for communication. In the days that followed, it was remarkable to hear Daryl reiterate the plan, ensuring we wouldn't get lost again. A truly memorable learning experience for both! And a reminder for me to be clearer in expectations.

That day at Costco reminded me how fragile our systems had become—how easily a missed signal could spiral into confusion. But it wasn't just stores and phones. Even the paths we once knew by heart were beginning to feel unfamiliar.

# Off Course

In July 2025, while riding his trike around Lake Nokomis, the sun reflected off the water, a gentle breeze brushed our cheeks and geese crossed the path. After one round, Daryl asked if we should go around again. My response was, "Whatever you want to do."

As we glide into the second loop, halfway around the curve, I noticed his right shoulder slump. He struggled to sit upright and—click—his feet slipped free of the pedals. The trike wobbled toward the grass. Before I can re-strap him, three teens in neon vests—park volunteers—hear my shout and sprint over. In seconds, they hoist Daryl upright, snap his shoes back into the clips, and offer quick words of encouragement. He nods, determination flickering in his eyes, and we roll on.

A quarter mile later, the path narrows. Daryl's body drifts right again, the trike fishtails off the path—and slides down an incline landing in the grass on its side, helmet skidding, a few irritated spots on his head from the helmet.

My heart hammers as I scramble down to him. Relieved he was stunned but unhurt. Several bystanders rushed over to help as the trike tipped onto its side. After a quick discussion, it was decided that I would ride my e-trike the half-mile back home to get the car, while the others stayed behind to watch over Daryl. As I started the quick ride back home, my thoughts raced faster than the e-trike. I replayed the fall over and over in my head, wondering if Daryl might be more seriously hurt than he'd let on. Every bump in the path made me anxious to get back to him. I pushed the trike as fast as I could, hoping the others would be able to keep him calm and safe until I returned with the car. I kept telling myself he was in good care.

When home, my son, Brian, was in the garage. "What's going on?" He asked. "Daryl fell off his trike, I replied. Brian asked where and I was unable to be helpful with location. Quickly, he blurted, "I will check Find My Friends and meet you at the lake-now!"

When I pull up in the car, Brian is already crouched beside Daryl, voice calm and firm:

"One... two... three... STAND!

One... two... three...MOVE!"

He counts again—sidestep, shuffle, forward—until Daryl reaches the van's open door. Each command cracked the freeze in his legs, each step a small victory.

Using a few firm, specific commands Brian guided Daryl get into the front passenger seat. Daryl climbed in and sank back with a relieved breath. Brian then hoisted the trike and stowed it in the back of the van.

At home, the stairlift hums him upstairs to his favorite recliner. He sinks into its cushions, eyes closed, relief softening his features.

The fall shook us both. It was a reminder that even familiar places could turn treacherous. But two weeks later, we returned—not because the fear had vanished, but because the courage had grown. And in that return, we found something unexpected.

# Tiny Triumphs

Two weeks later, the sun calls us back. Perpetually drifting right on his etrike, Daryl was teetering on the edge of the path again. My heart pounded. Every bump, every slight swerve, sent a jolt of fear. Parkinson's is a constant navigation, and right now, his tendency to favor the right was leading him into a dangerous dance with the edge of the path.

"Stay to the left! Stay to the left!" Periodically, I reminded him, switching my negative thoughts of fear, to how I value the special moments we share enjoying the beautiful scenery.

One lap. Then two. Three laps of tiny triumphs.

Studies suggest that people with LPD (Left-onset Parkinson's Disease) may exhibit a rightward visual field, meaning they have a tendency to perceive stimuli as shifted slightly to the right.

We had learned to navigate the falls, the missteps, the moments when Parkinson's rewrote the rules mid-journey. But surviving each episode wasn't enough. Something deeper was stirring—a shift from reacting to understanding, from bracing to embracing. And with that shift came a new kind of knowing, one rooted not in control, but in clarity.

# Chapter Twelve: The Shift from Surviving to Knowing

## Surrendering to What Matters

There comes a point in caregiving when the chaos doesn't stop—but your response to it changes. For me, that shift began not in a hospital or a crisis. It began on July 17, 2024, in a virtual session hosted by the Veteran's Support Group at the Los Angeles VA Medical Center. That afternoon, I logged in from my apartment, surrounded by other caregivers, guided by two facilitators whose calm wisdom cut through the noise.

"Parkinson's is a disease of deception," one of the presenters began, her voice steady and clear. Around the screen, heads nodded. We were all learning to read between the lines—what looked like stubbornness might be fear, what seemed like forgetfulness could be fatigue. That day, she introduced us to Self-Determination Theory, a framework that helped us understand how to support our loved ones without taking over.

- **Autonomy:** "Let them choose," she said. "Involve them in decisions." I thought of our morning routine. Instead of saying, It's time to go triking, I'd started asking, Should we go triking this morning or after dinner? That small shift gave Daryl a sense of control, even on days when Parkinson's felt like it was calling the shots.

- **Competence:** "Break down tasks. Offer cues, not commands." She demonstrated with a smile: When standing up from the chair, remember—nose over toes. It was gentle, empowering. I'd seen how Daryl responded better to reminders than instructions. It preserved his dignity.
- **Connection:** "Use memory tools as a team," she said. We'd already started setting pill reminders on his iPhone, using calendar alerts and alarms. It wasn't just about managing medication—it was about staying connected, sharing responsibility.
- **Redirect:** "Routines and visual cues matter," she emphasized. In our apartment, sticky notes had become part of the décor. One on the bathroom mirror simply said LOUD—a reminder for Daryl to project his voice. Another near the bed prompted him to do his core exercises first thing in the morning. These cues weren't nagging—they were anchors.

That afternoon, I signed off feeling steadier. The theory wasn't just academic—it was a lifeline. It gave me language for what we were already doing, and tools for what we hadn't yet tried. Most of all, it reminded me that caregiving isn't about fixing—it's about partnering, adapting, and honoring the person you love.

Before that day, I thought caregiving was about endurance—about showing up, staying strong, and holding everything together. But what I learned in that virtual circle, with her voice guiding us through the fog, was that caregiving is also about surrender. Not to the disease, but to the relationship. To the possibility that even in decline, there is dignity. Even in uncertainty, there is choice. And even in the smallest routines, there is love.

That afternoon's insights didn't just shift my mindset—they reshaped our routines. One of the most immediate challenges we faced was nighttime mobility. What seemed like a simple struggle to turn over in bed became a window into how Parkinson's was stealing comfort, autonomy, and rest. So we asked for help—and found new ways to adapt.

## Wrestling with the Sheets: When Turning Over Turns Into a Battle

It started with the nights. Daryl would wake up, restless and uncomfortable, trying to shift positions but unable to turn over. Eventually, he'd give up and shuffle to his recliner, hoping for relief. I'd hear the rustling, the sighs, the quiet frustration. Sometimes he'd call for me—not loudly, just a soft "Can you help me?" And I'd go, lifting his feet, guiding his hand, trying not to strain my back.

I didn't realize how much effort it took him until I saw it through his physical therapist's eyes. She called it "bed mobility impairment"—a common challenge for people with Parkinson's. The stiffness, the slowness, the tremors—they all conspire against the simple act of turning over in bed. It's not just discomfort. It's a loss of autonomy.

We asked for help. She laid him on a firm training bed and watched. Then she taught us a series of exercises—gentle movements to loosen his trunk, activate his legs, and prepare his body for the effort of getting up.

Here's what she showed us:

- **Lower Trunk Rotation**
  With knees bent and feet flat, Daryl slowly rotates his legs side to side. It's like coaxing his body to remember how to move.
- **Supine Heel Slides**
  One heel at a time, sliding toward the buttocks, then back. A quiet rhythm.
- **Supine March**
  Lifting each leg, one at a time, knees bent, feet flat. It looks simple, but it's a workout.

Then came the technique for getting up:

- Sit with knees toward the end of the bed.
- Hips near the pillow.
- Bend one knee.
- Punch with the far arm—yes, punch. She held out her hands and had him punch with intent.
- Prop onto the elbow.
- Punch again to rise.

It's not elegant, but it works. And it gives him a sense of control.

We made changes at home too. Raised the head of the bed. Added a rail. Swapped our sheets for ones with a satin center panel—smooth enough to glide, but not so slippery that he'd slide out. The therapist warned us about full satin or silk sheets. Too dangerous.

These small adjustments—exercises, techniques, fabric choices—are our nightly rituals now. They don't fix everything, but they help. And in this journey, every bit of help matters.

These nighttime challenges—restlessness, discomfort, the struggle to turn over—were just one part of the larger picture. The support group didn't just offer tips for sleep; it gave me a new way to think about tomorrow. About reclaiming rhythm, purpose, and hope.

## Walking Towards Tomorrow

One of the facilitators also reminded us that tomorrow often never comes unless we give it shape. He urged us to craft SMART goals—specific, measurable, achievable, results-oriented, time-bound. So I vowed to walk two hours around Lake Nokomis at least four days a week, with a health aide at Daryl's side. At my own pace, pausing on benches to drink in the sunrise. Each loop becomes a promise—a small victory against the night and a step toward reclaiming our rhythms.

I didn't leave that support group with all the answers. But I left with something better: a new lens. One that helped me see Daryl not just as someone I needed to care for, but as someone I could care with.

Setting goals gave me direction. Walking around Lake Nokomis became a ritual of renewal—a way to reclaim rhythm and breathe through the chaos. But even as I moved forward, I couldn't ignore what lingered behind.

# The Loss of "Us"

I stood at the garage door, helmet in hand, ready for our three rounds circling Lake Nokomis—only to recall how our 30-mile rides had slipped beyond reach. The morning air felt empty as our trike tires echoed a quiet hum against the pavement. In that hush, I tasted grief for the person he once was and the adventures we lost.

That morning at the garage door marked more than the loss of a ride—it marked the loss of a rhythm we once shared. But grief, I learned, doesn't just take things away. It also opens space. Space to see the person in front of me not as who he was, but as who he is now. And that shift changed everything.

# Embracing the Person Before

Parkinson's doesn't just change muscles; it reshapes identity. I learned to show up differently—lean in when he struggles to button his shirt, slide my hand into his to steady his step, sit beside him in the quiet he once filled with conversation. Instead of asking, "Why can't we do the trips we planned?" I started asking, "How can I be here for him now?"

Learning to be present in the now softened my expectations. It also deepened our connection. As Parkinson's reshaped our routines, it reshaped our intimacy too—not by erasing it, but by inviting us to rediscover it in quieter, more tender ways.

## Rediscovering Intimacy

Parkinson's changed how we touched, how we expressed desire, how we felt close. The physical act became less central—but the emotional and sensory connection grew deeper. We learned to be open, sensitive, and experimental. A sneak-up hug in the kitchen. A kiss on the shoulder while folding laundry. Back scratches, hand-holding, shared warmth under the covers. These became our love language. Sometimes, Daryl whispered, "I thank God every night for you. I love you." And in that moment, I felt more cherished than any grand romantic gesture could offer.

We didn't lose intimacy. We reshaped it.

That rediscovery of closeness became the foundation for something even more surprising: joy. Not the kind we used to chase on long bike rides or weekend getaways, but the kind that lives in the everyday—in tacos, in footsteps, in whispered thanks.

## Finding Joy in Our Backyard

Like Dorothy discovering that happiness wasn't "over the rainbow," I began hunting for ruby-slipper moments at home—a plate of tacos eaten with our friends, the soft thump of his sneakers above our stairs as he tries to keep his balance. Each "thank you" he whispers, every unexpected hug, feels like gold.

Caregiving became a physical, intimate dance of attention and tenderness. Without Parkinson's, I might never have learned that presence—just being beside someone—is the greatest gift. In the steady rhythm of shared routines, we discovered a new kind of control: the power to choose love over loss every single day.

*"I didn't know then what caregiving would ask of me. But I knew I wouldn't walk away. Love, in its truest form, doesn't flinch—it adapts."*

Joy gave me strength. But strength alone wasn't enough. I needed tools—ways to stay grounded when the days grew heavy, when the nights stretched long, when the questions had no easy answers. So I began building my caregiver's toolbox.

# The Caregiver's Toolbox

These moments—of falling, of waking at 2 a.m., of choosing love over loss—taught me more than any manual ever could. But I still wish I'd had one. A guide for the emotional terrain, the mental gymnastics, the quiet recalibrations. So I began building one. Not just for me, but for anyone walking this path. What follows isn't theory—it's lived experience. These are the strategies I reach for when the ground shifts. My caregiver toolbox.

I needed tools. Not just logistical plans, but emotional strategies. Ways to stay grounded, clear-headed, and compassionate—even when my heart was racing and my patience was fraying.

I began collecting techniques like lifelines:

- Getting Rid of ANTs (Automatic Negative Thoughts)
- Deep Breathing
- Mindfulness
- Boundaries
- Let Them (the art of letting go)
- Stress Relief rituals—walks, music, nature
- Speak from the "I"
- From Wishful Thinking to Purposeful Action
- Compassion for the Caregiver
- Solving Problems with Clarity
- Compassion
- Journaling—Writing Through the Storm
- Respite—The Gift of Stepping Away

Each one became a thread in the net I now carry with me. I wish I'd known them earlier. I wish someone had handed me a manual for the emotional terrain of caregiving. But maybe this memoir can be that manual—for someone else.

I didn't arrive at this toolbox overnight. It was built slowly, through trial and error, through moments of grace and grit. Each tool was forged in the fire of experience—some discovered in desperation, others in quiet revelation. They didn't just help me survive; they helped me understand. They became the scaffolding for a new kind of knowing.

Knowing that caregiving is not a role—it's a relationship.

Knowing that resilience is not just bouncing back—it's growing forward.

Knowing that love, when stretched across uncertainty, becomes something sacred.

This next section is not a prescription. It's a companion. A collection of strategies that sustained me—and might sustain you. Part II is where the memoir becomes a map. Let's walk it together.

PART II

# THE CAREGIVER'S TOOLBOX: STRATEGIES THAT SUSTAIN ME

*Lived practices that restore balance, clarity, and grace*
*"You can't stop the waves, but you can learn to surf."*
**—Jon Kabat-Zinn**

# Strategy One: Getting Rid of ANTs: Reclaiming Your Thoughts

*"If you realized how powerful your thoughts are, you would never think a negative thought."*
**—Peace Pilgrim**
*This strategy changed how I speak to myself. It's not just about thoughts—it's about freedom.*

## What Are ANTs?

Caregiving often feels like a storm of emotions—frustration, sadness, guilt, even resentment. But beneath those feelings are thoughts. And when those thoughts go unchecked, they can spiral into what psychologists call ANTs: Automatic Negative Thoughts. These are the reflexive, often distorted beliefs that creep in when we're overwhelmed.

The concept of automatic negative thoughts was first introduced by Dr. Aaron Beck, a pioneer of cognitive therapy. He showed how our internal dialogue can distort reality and fuel emotional distress. Later, psychiatrist Dr. Daniel Amen coined the term "ANTs," likening these thoughts to mental pests—uninvited, persistent, and often irrational. His metaphor helped make the concept more accessible, especially for those navigating stress.

Understanding how thoughts shape feelings—and how feelings shape actions—was a turning point for me. I learned that I could catch unhelpful thoughts and gently shift them into something more constructive. It wasn't about denying reality. It was about choosing a lens that helped me cope, not crumble.

## Three Common ANTs

### Extreme Thinking

This is all-or-nothing thinking—no middle ground.

*"I'm devastated that Daryl has Parkinson's. He won't be able to clean the bathrooms."*

Now I say:
*"I'm devastated that Daryl has Parkinson's, but he can still help me make the bed."*

That small shift doesn't erase the grief. But it softens it. It reminds me that loss and contribution can coexist.

### "Should" Statements

*"Daryl should clean up his own mess."*

Now I say:
*"Daryl can clean up his own mess."*

These thoughts often lead to frustration—not because they're wrong, but because they're rigid. Parkinson's doesn't follow rules. And expecting others to meet our internal standards can set us up for disappointment. Replacing "should" with "can" or "might" opens space for compassion.

**Not Finding the Positive**

*"Our daughter-in-law can't take Daryl to work out on Saturday."*

Now I say:
*"She can't come Saturday, but she cares enough to come Sunday."*

It's easy to focus on what's missing. But shifting our gaze to what's offered—even if it's imperfect—can change everything.

# A Personal Reframe

When Daryl and I were downsizing for our move to Minneapolis, I felt a wave of anger. He refused to part with his old briefcases—relics of a life that felt long gone. My first thought: Why can't he just let go? But then I paused. I reframed: If he's not ready, we'll pack them. He can store them under the TV until he is.

That single shift turned my anger into calm. It wasn't about the briefcases. It was about honoring his process.

# Why It Matters

Unprocessed anger doesn't just live in the mind—it settles in the body. It can cause digestive issues, headaches, tension, sleep disturbances, anxiety, and depression. I used to stuff my anger until it exploded—often over something unrelated. I didn't know I could choose my thoughts. Now I do.

# Tools That Help

- **Thought-stopping**: When a negative spiral begins, say "Stop" out loud or in your mind. Then breathe.
- **Reframing**: Ask, Is there another way to see this? Even a small shift can ease the emotional load.
- **Journaling**: Write the thought. Then write a kinder version. Let your pen be your witness.
- **Compassion**: Celebrate what you did today, not what you didn't. You're doing enough.
- **Connection**: Share your feelings with someone who understands. Support groups can be lifelines.
- **Patience**: Noticing ANTs takes practice. But noticing is the first step. And every step counts.

# Closing Reflection

*Getting rid of ANTs isn't about perfection—it's about permission. Permission to pause. Permission to reframe. Permission to speak to yourself with the same kindness you offer others.*

Each time you catch an ANT and choose a gentler thought, you reclaim a piece of your peace. You remind yourself that caregiving doesn't have to be a battlefield of the mind. It can be a practice of grace.

**Thoughts are not facts. They're invitations. And you get to decide which ones you accept.**

Once I began noticing my thoughts, I realized my body needed support too. I found that breathing, slow intentional breaths—helped ground me.

# Strategy Two: Breathing Through the Storm

*"Feelings come and go like clouds in a windy sky. Conscious breathing is my anchor."*
**—Thich Nhat Hanh**

## What Is Deep Breathing?

Deep breathing is more than a relaxation technique—it's a way to reclaim calm when the world feels overwhelming. It activates the parasympathetic nervous system, which helps the body relax, lowers stress hormones, and increases oxygen to the brain and muscles. It's simple, portable, and powerful.

Though breathwork has ancient roots in yoga and meditation, it was teachers like Thich Nhat Hanh who helped bring conscious breathing into everyday life. His gentle wisdom reminded us that each breath is a chance to return to ourselves. In modern psychology, deep breathing is now recognized as a foundational tool for emotional regulation and stress relief.

*Here's how I practice it:*

- **Find a comfortable spot**—bed, chair, floor, or even a

patch of grass.

- **Place one hand** on your chest and one on your belly.
- **Inhale slowly** through your nose, feeling your belly rise.
- **Exhale gently** through pursed lips, letting your belly fall.
- **Repeat** for a few minutes, focusing only on your breath.

## A Personal Reframe

When Daryl's snoring wakes me in the middle of the night, I nudge him gently and try to return to sleep. If I can't, I lie on my back and begin my breathwork:

- **Inhale** to a count of 4.
- **Hold** for 4.
- **Exhale** for 4.

I focus on the rhythm, sometimes pairing it with a breath prayer:

- **Inhale:** "*Come to me*"
- **Hold:** (silent pause)
- **Exhale:** "*and I will give you rest.*" (Matthew 11:28)

*It's not just about falling back asleep—it's about finding peace in the pause.*

# Breathing in Nature

On walks around Lake Nokomis, I often pause on a bench, close my eyes, and take a few deep breaths as the wind rustles through the trees. *It's a moment of stillness in a life that rarely stops.*

# Breathing in Motion

I've woven breathwork into my daily neck and core exercises.
*For example:*
**Neck Stretch**

- Left hand on belly, right hand on shoulder.
- Face turns right. Feel the stretch.
- Inhale to 5, exhale. Repeat 3 times.
- Repeat three sets, then switch sides.


**Core Stretch (after Clam Shell)**

- Lying on my side, hands clasped behind my head.
- Left elbow grounded, right elbow stretching upward.
- Inhale to 5, hold, exhale to 5—Repeat three times.
- Rest. Repeat three sets. Switch sides.

*These movements, paired with breath, help me feel centered and strong.*

## Tools That Help

- **Notice:** Your belly should rise more than your chest—like a balloon inflating.
- **Count:** I often use 4-4-4 or 5-5-5 rhythms depending on the exercise.
- **Concentrate:** Feel your breath. Let it guide you.
- **Relax:** Let tension leave your body with each exhale.
- **Visualize:** Imagine breathing in peace, breathing out stress.
- **Be Patient:** If you feel dizzy, slow down. Gentleness matters.
- **Practice Daily:** Even a few minutes a day can make a difference.
- **Use at Point of Need:** Breath is always with you. Use it anytime, anywhere!

## Closing Reflection

These tools don't erase the hard days. But they soften them. They remind me that I'm not just reacting—I'm choosing. And in that choice, I find strength, clarity, and love. If you're reading this, I hope you find your own toolbox. Fill it slowly. Use it often. And know that you're not alone.

Breath was my anchor. But presence—moment by moment—became my lifeline.

# Strategy Three: Mindfulness, The Art of Noticing

*"Mindfulness isn't difficult. We just need to remember to do it."*
**—Sharon Salzberg**

## What Is Mindfulness?

Mindfulness is the practice of being fully present—aware of your thoughts, sensations, and emotions without judgment. It's not about clearing your mind or escaping reality. It's about anchoring yourself in it. For caregivers, mindfulness can be a lifeline. It helps us respond instead of react, soften instead of snap, and find peace in the middle of the storm.

While mindfulness has deep roots in Buddhist tradition, it was Dr. Jon Kabat-Zinn who helped bring it into Western medicine. In the 1970s, he developed Mindfulness-Based Stress Reduction (MBSR), a program that showed how present-moment awareness could reduce pain, anxiety, and emotional overwhelm. His work helped bridge ancient wisdom with modern science—making mindfulness a practical tool for healing and resilience.

# A Personal Reframe

Each afternoon, when Daryl's home health aide arrives, I lace up my shoes and head to Lake Nokomis. The path is familiar, but never the same. I hear the crunch of leaves beneath my feet, watch mother geese nudge their goslings through the grass, smell the sweet smoke of hamburgers on a nearby grill. The breeze brushes my skin as I walk past the shoreline. A mosquito bite itches on my leg—and I let it go.

At home, I practice mindfulness in quieter ways. I notice the craving for monster cookies and remind myself I have control. I savor the warmth of hot chocolate, the softness of melted marshmallows. I feel the comfort of a warm compress over my eyes at night. I breathe deeply. I let emotions rise and fall like waves. I don't chase them. I don't fight them. I simply witness them.

Mindfulness isn't a ritual—it's a rhythm. A way of being present, anytime, anywhere.

# Why It Matters

Mindfulness enhances every part of our well-being:

- **Mental Health**
  - Reduces stress and anxiety
  - Fosters self-acceptance
  - Helps us respond thoughtfully to emotions

- Deepens understanding of our thoughts and behaviors
- Improves focus and clarity
- **Physical Health**
  - Promotes better sleep
  - Lowers blood pressure
  - Helps shift attention away from pain
  - Supports immune function
- **Relationships**
  - Builds empathy and compassion
  - Encourages listening
  - Improves communication and emotional regulation

# Tools That Help

## Mindful Practices

- Meditation – even five minutes can reset your day
- Movement – yoga, walking, biking with awareness
- Mindful Eating – savoring flavors, textures, and temperature
- Active Listening – being fully present when someone speaks

## Digital & Media Tools

- Apps – Calm, Insight Timer, Headspace

- Websites – mindful.org, The Mental Health Foundation
- Books – Authors like Thich Nhat Hanh (Peace Is Every Step) and Dan Harris (10% Happier)

## Sensory Anchors

- Candles, incense, singing bowls
- A small altar or dedicated space
- Nature sounds or soft music

## Community

- Mindfulness classes
- Support groups for caregivers
- Guided meditations with others

# Closing Reflection

I often found myself ruminating on the past or worrying about the future. Mindfulness helped me stay grounded, gently guiding me to focus on the present moment without judgment.

Mindfulness doesn't erase the hard parts of caregiving. But it gives them space. It allows us to breathe through the tension, to notice the beauty tucked between the burdens, and to remember that presence is its own kind of healing. Every time I choose to notice instead of numb, I reclaim a piece of myself. With clarity came courage. I began to see where I ended and where caregiving began.

# Strategy Four: Setting Boundaries Without Guilt

*"You can't pour from an empty cup. Setting boundaries isn't selfish—it's survival."*
**—Author Unknown**

## What Are Boundaries?

Boundaries are the invisible lines that protect your time, energy, and emotional well-being. They're not walls—they're gates. They help you decide what you can offer, when you need to step back, and how to preserve your own health while caring for someone else.

As a caregiver, boundaries are often tested. Parkinson's doesn't respect schedules. It doesn't ask permission. But that doesn't mean you have to say yes to everything—or carry the weight alone.

In recent years, therapists and authors like Dr. Henry Cloud, Dr. John Townsend, and Nedra Glover Tawwab have helped bring boundary-setting into everyday conversations. Their work reminds us that boundaries aren't barriers—they're bridges to healthier relationships and sustainable caregiving.

# A Personal Reframe

In the early days of caregiving, I said yes to everything. Every appointment, every errand, every emotional need. I thought that was love. But over time, I realized that love without limits leads to burnout.

When Daryl's care team expanded, I found myself coordinating helpers, managing medications, and still trying to keep our home running. One day, I caught myself snapping at a friend—not because of her, but because I hadn't taken a moment for myself in weeks.

*That was the wake-up call. I started small:*

- I blocked out two hours each week for a solo walk around Lake Nokomis.
- I let go of guilt when I said, *"I can't do that today."*
- I posted our care schedule on the fridge and stopped answering last-minute texts that disrupted our rhythm.

*Each boundary was a breath of fresh air. Not a rejection—but a recalibration.*

# Why It Matters

Setting boundaries helps you:

- **Prevent burnout** and emotional exhaustion

- **Protect your physical health**
- **Preserve relationships** by reducing resentment
- **Create space** for joy, rest, and renewal
- **Model healthy limits** for others in your care circle

*Boundaries aren't barriers—they're bridges to sustainability.*

# Tools That Help

- **The Pause Button:** Before saying yes, pause. Ask: *"Do I have the bandwidth for this?"*
- **The "No" That Honors You:**
  - *"I wish I could, but I need to rest."*
  - *"Let's revisit this next week."*
  - *"I'm not available right now, but here's what I can offer."*
- **The Schedule That Speaks for You:** Post your routine. Let it be your voice when you're too tired to explain.
- **The Guilt Reframe:** Guilt says, *"I'm not doing enough."* Boundaries say, *"I'm doing what's sustainable."*
- **The Trusted Circle:** Share your limits with people who respect them. Let them help hold the line.

# Closing Reflection

Boundaries aren't selfish. They're sacred. They allow you to show up with presence instead of resentment, with energy instead of exhaustion. Every time you say *"not now,"* you're saying *"yes"* to your own well-being—and that's a gift to everyone you care for.

Some boundaries are firm. Others are soft. And some are simply about letting go.

# Strategy Five: Let Them Be, Let Yourself Breathe

*"Letting go doesn't mean giving up. It means making space—for peace, for dignity, for love."*
**—Vincent Woodard**

## What Is the "Let Them" Mindset?

Popularized by Mel Robbins, the "Let Them" theory is a shift in mindset that invites us to release the need to control others—their choices, reactions, or pace. It's not about indifference. It's about respect. It's about choosing to focus on what we can control: our own thoughts, actions, and emotional responses.

In caregiving, this shift is profound. It allows us to stop wrestling with what we wish were different—and start honoring what is.

## A Personal Reframe

Daryl loves his old shirts. They're soft, familiar, and worn with memory. I used to nudge him toward buying new ones.

Now, I let him wear what he loves. It's one less battle—and one more moment of peace.

He struggles with his CPAP machine. Says he can't breathe. I used to remind, coax, worry. Now, I let him decide. I can't control his comfort. But I can control my response.

When tax season came, I worried about his cognitive decline. I feared mistakes. But this year, I let him take the lead. Slowly, methodically, he worked through the forms. It wasn't perfect—but it was dignified. And that mattered more.

*Letting go didn't mean stepping away. It meant stepping back—just enough to let him stand.*

## Why It Matters

*The "Let Them" mindset helps us:*

- **Reduce** anxiety and emotional exhaustion
- **Honor** autonomy and dignity
- **Establish** healthy boundaries
- **Focus** on what's within our control
- **Respond** with grace instead of resistance

It's not passive—it's powerful.

# Tools That Help

- **Acknowledge Reality:**
    - You can't control others' thoughts, feelings, or actions.
    - You can control your response.
- **Manage Your Emotions:**
    - Notice what triggers frustration.
    - Write it down.
    - *"Is this mine to fix?" "Or theirs to feel?"*
- **Identify Your Values:**
    - What matters most: peace, dignity, connection?
    - What choice can you make that honors those values?
- **Say "Let Me...":**
    - *"Let me choose calm."*
    - *"Let me focus on what I can do."*
    - *"Let me be present, not perfect."*

# Closing Reflection

Letting go isn't easy. But it's freeing. It allows us to stop micromanaging moments and start living them. It reminds us that love isn't control—it's compassion. And sometimes, the most powerful thing we can do is simply let them.

*"You can always choose what you think, say, or do in response to other people, the world around you, or the emotions rising up inside of you. That's the source of all your power."*
**—Mel Robbins, The Let Them Theory**

Letting go created space. In that space, I began to build rituals that restored me.

# Strategy Six: Rituals That Restore Me

*"Ritual is the passageway of the soul into the Infinite."*
**—Algernon Blackwood**

## What Are Stress Relief Rituals?

Stress relief rituals are the small, intentional acts that help me reset—physically, emotionally, and spiritually. They're not luxuries. They're lifelines. Whether it's a warm bath, a walk in nature, a favorite song, or a quiet prayer, these rituals help me reconnect with myself when caregiving pulls me in every direction.

They don't fix everything. But they soften the edges.

## A Personal Reframe

Some evenings, I slip into a warm bath infused with essential oils. The scent of lavender or eucalyptus fills the room, and my muscles begin to unclench. It's not just about hygiene—it's about healing.

On walks with my friend, Trudi, around Lake Nokomis,

we listen to birdsong and share our hopes and worries. The breeze, the rhythm of our steps, the quiet companionship—it all soothes my nervous system.

You don't need a lake to feel this kind of calm. Your "Lake Nokomis" might be a quiet park, a tree-lined street, or even a cozy corner of your home. What matters is finding a space where you feel safe, grounded, and able to connect—with yourself or someone you trust. Try noticing where your body feels most at ease, and return there often.

Each morning begins with a devotional. Scripture replaces anxious thoughts with hope. It's a moment of stillness before the day begins—a sacred pause.

And then there's music. Bobby Bare's "500 Miles Away from Home," "Streets of Baltimore," "Tequila Sheila"—songs from the 70s and 80s when Daryl was stationed in Germany, waiting for me to join him. These melodies carry memory, connection, and comfort. Roy Orbison's "Oh, Pretty Woman" and "Blue Bayou" fill the room with nostalgia and joy. For Daryl, they're reminders of a younger version of us. For me, they're medicine.

## Why It Matters

*Stress relief rituals support well-being in powerful ways:*

- **Physically**
  - Activate the parasympathetic nervous system
  - Lower heart rate and blood pressure

- ◦ Relax tense muscles
- **Emotionally**

  - ◦ Release dopamine and serotonin
  - ◦ Shift focus from stress to presence
  - ◦ Promote mindfulness and emotional regulation
- **Relationally**

  - ◦ Strengthen connection
  - ◦ Build trust and empathy
  - ◦ Create shared moments of peace

# Tools That Help

**Physical Comforts**

- Essential oils
- Scented candles
- Cozy clothing
- Bath milk and massage tools
- Eye packs and wraps
- Music therapy and visualization

**Sacred Spaces**

- A quiet corner with soft light
- A favorite bench in nature
- A devotional nook with meaningful objects

# Closing Reflection

Rituals are more than routines. They're acts of care—toward ourselves, toward others, toward the moment we're in. They help us move through anxiety, reconnect with meaning, and remember who we are beneath the stress.

Start small. Maybe it's brewing coffee in a favorite mug while watching the sunrise. Maybe it's lighting a candle before bed. Whatever it is, let it be yours. Let it be enough.

As I found ways to soothe myself, I also learned how to speak for myself—with honesty and grace.

# Strategy Seven: Speak from the "I": Communicating with Clarity and Compassion

*"Speak your truth, but keep your heart open."*
**—Author Unknown**

## What Are "I Statements"?

"I statements" are a way of expressing your feelings, needs, and boundaries without blame. Instead of saying, "You never listen to me," you say, "I feel unheard when I try to share something important." The shift is subtle—but powerful. It invites understanding instead of defensiveness.

As a caregiver, I've learned that "I statements" help me stay grounded in my own experience while still honoring Daryl's. They allow me to communicate clearly, kindly, and effectively—even when emotions run high.

This approach is rooted in assertiveness training and was later refined through the work of psychologist Marshall Rosenberg, who developed Nonviolent Communication (NVC). His framework emphasized speaking from personal experience while staying connected to empathy and compassion—especially in moments of conflict.

## A Personal Reframe

When Daryl forgets to take his medication, my instinct used to be frustration:*"You forgot again!"*

**Now I say:**

*"I feel worried when your medication schedule gets off track. Can we look at it together?"*

Sometimes we explore setting reminders on his iPhone or our Google Nest.

When I'm overwhelmed by the day's demands, I don't lash out.

**I say:**

*"I need a few quiet minutes to recharge. I'll be more present afterward."*

When discussing respite care, I used to say, "I *need a break.*" But that felt vague and reactive.

**Now I say:**

*"I need two hours each afternoon to take a brisk walk around Lake Nokomis. Taking time for myself helps me be a better partner."*

That opened a thoughtful conversation about Daryl's preferences—timing, days, and caregiver gender.

When advocating for consistent care routines, I didn't say, *"This schedule is a mess."*

**I said:**

"I need one caregiver five days a week, two hours a day. That consistency helps calm Daryl's anxiety. I understand scheduling is complex. I'm willing to be flexible."

That clarity led to real options—and real relief.

When my lower back began aching from lifting the foot soak container, I didn't say, "I'm breaking my back!"

**I said:**

"I need your helper to take over the foot soak routine so I can protect my back for other caregiving tasks."

Even small moments benefit from this shift. When the oven is left on, I don't accuse.

**I say:**

"I get worried when the oven is left on. I'd like to find a solution so we both feel safe."

Each time I speak from the "I," I feel more grounded. And Daryl feels more respected.

# Why It Matters

"I statements" help caregivers:

- **Express** emotions without blame
- **Reduce** conflict and defensiveness
- **Clarify** needs and boundaries
- **Strengthen** trust and empathy
- **Model** respectful communication

They're especially helpful when navigating cognitive changes, emotional shifts, or logistical stress.

## Tools That Help

**The Formula**

I feel **[emotion]** when **[situation]** because **[reason]**. I need/would like **[request]**.

**Example**

*"I feel anxious when we're late for appointments because it's hard to reschedule. I'd like us to leave ten minutes earlier."*

**Practice Prompts**

- *"I feel..."*
- *"I need..."*
- *"I would appreciate..."*
- *"I'm struggling with..."*
- *"I'd like to find a solution together..."*

**Tips**

- Use a calm tone and open body language
- Focus on your experience, not their behavior
- Pair with active listening
- Write statements down first, if needed. That's how I practiced.

# Closing Reflection

Finding your voice as a caregiver isn't about being loud—it's about being clear. "I statements" help you speak from the heart, advocate for your needs, and build bridges instead of walls. They remind us that communication isn't just about words—it's about connection, dignity, and the quiet courage to ask for what you need.

Naming my needs was powerful. But naming wasn't enough—I needed a plan.

# Strategy Eight: From Wishful Thinking to Purposeful Action

*"A goal without a plan is just a wish."*
**—Antoine de Saint-Exupéry**

## What Is a SMART Goal?

SMART goals are a way to turn intentions into action. They help caregivers move from "I should" to "I will"—with clarity, structure, and purpose. Each goal includes five key elements:

- **Specific** – What exactly do you want to accomplish?
- **Measurable** – How will you track progress?
- **Achievable** – Is it realistic and within reach?
- **Relevant** – Why does it matter to you?
- **Time-Bound** – When will it be completed?

SMART goals don't just organize your day—they organize your mind.

The SMART framework was first introduced in 1981 by George T. Doran in a management journal, but its clarity and usefulness quickly spread beyond business. Today, it's used in education, therapy, and personal development—including caregiving. For me, SMART goals became a way to reclaim agency in a world that often felt unpredictable.

# A Personal Reframe

Instead of saying, "*I need more exercise,*" I created a SMART goal:

"*I will walk around Lake Nokomis for two hours a day, four days a week—Monday, Tuesday, Wednesday, and Friday—while Rahsaan is with Daryl. I'll highlight each walk on my calendar for one month to track my progress and improve my health.*"

**Let's break it down:**

- **Specific** – Walk two hours a day
- **Measurable** – Four days a week
- **Achievable** – Fits into my caregiving schedule
- **Relevant** – Supports my physical and emotional health
- **Time-Bound** – One month

Other goals followed:

- "*I will add each appointment to both Daryl's calendar and my iPhone immediately after it's scheduled, and confirm the week's schedule every Sunday night.*"
- "*Rahsaan, I need the apartment vacuumed every Friday*

*while Daryl's feet are soaking."*

These goals aren't just tasks—they're commitments. They help me stay focused, communicate clearly, and feel a sense of progress in a life that often feels unpredictable.

## Why It Matters

- **Eliminate vagueness** and indecision
- **Prioritize self-care** and household needs
- **Communicate clearly** with care teams
- **Track progress** and celebrate small wins
- **Adapt** to changing circumstances with flexibility

*They turn overwhelm into order—and intention into impact.*

## Tools That Help

- **Write it down** – Clarity begins on paper
- **Use your calendar** – Schedule each step
- **Reflect weekly** – What worked? What didn't?
- **Modify as needed** – Goals are living things
- **Celebrate progress** – Even small steps count

# Closing Reflection

SMART goals don't just help you get things done—they help you feel more grounded, more capable, and more in control. They remind you that even in the chaos of caregiving, you can choose your direction. So start small. Be specific. And when life shifts, let your goals shift with it. No guilt—just growth.

Even with goals, I stumbled. That's when I learned the most important strategy of all: compassion—for myself.

# Strategy Nine: Compassion for the Caregiver—Grace, Self-forgiveness, and Emotional Renewal

*"Talk to yourself like someone you love."*
**—Brené Brown**

## What Is Compassion for the Caregiver?

Caregiving demands deep wells of patience, strength, and love—but too often, caregivers forget to extend those same gifts to themselves. Compassion for the caregiver means learning to forgive your own missteps, offer yourself grace, and create space for emotional renewal. It's not indulgence—it's survival.

# A Personal Reframe

I grew up in a family where pleasing others was the gold standard. I chased perfection, believing that anything less would disappoint those around me. Over time, I internalized a chorus of critical voices that chipped away at my self-worth. Here are the categories of inner critics I carried with me:

- **Perfectionist—the relentless taskmaster who insists nothing you do is ever enough**
  - *"You should not make a mistake."*
  - *"You should not get an A-."*
  - *"You should not ask for help."*
- **Guilt—the emotional punisher who convinces you that everything is your fault**
  - *"She will never forgive you."*
  - *"You are not kind."*
  - *"You do not deserve to be loved."*
- **Inner Control—the enforcer who tried to keep you "in line"**
  - *"Shame on you."*
  - *"Don't try that."*
  - *"You have no self-control."*
- **Self-Doubt—the underminer who questions your abilities and worth**
  - *"Why try out? You'll fail."*
  - *"There's no point in doing that."*

- ◦ *"Your red hair looks ugly."*
- **Conforming—the people-pleaser who pushes you to blend in and avoid judgment**
  - ◦ *"Do what they want you to do."*
  - ◦ *"What will she think?"*
  - ◦ *"Don't do that—you'll look weird."*

Now, when my brain starts spinning those old tapes, I pause. I say or think, "STOP," and I replace the noise with affirmations that speak truth and kindness:

- *"I am who I am. There is no one like me."*
- *"I am worthy of kindness."*
- *"I am enough just as I am."*
- *"I forgive myself for my mistakes. I am human."*
- *"I am worthy of caring for myself."*
- *"I am strong."*

## Why It Matters

- **Eliminate vagueness** and indecision
- **Prioritize self-care** and household needs
- **Communicate clearly** with care teams
- **Track progress** and celebrate small wins
- **Adapt** to changing circumstances with flexibility

*They turn overwhelm into order—and intention into impact.*

# Tools That Help

**Practical ways to cultivate self-compassion:**

- **Replace harsh self-talk** with respectful, affirming language
- **Use daily positive affirmations**
- **Accept imperfections** as part of being human
- **Practice deep breathing** to calm the nervous system
- **Set and honor healthy boundaries**
- **Engage in mindfulness and guided meditations**
- **Journal** to explore your reflections and emotional shifts
- **Write a letter** to yourself about the part you want to heal
- **Nurture relationships** that uplift and support

# Closing Reflection

Self-sabotage is a quiet thief—it steals joy, confidence, and peace. But we can choose to stop being our own worst enemy. Happiness begins with self-acceptance. Mistakes are not failures—they're proof that we're trying, learning, and growing.

Letting go of what we cannot control, and embracing what we can, opens the door to grace. Taking time to rest and renew isn't selfish—it's sacred. Change takes time. Trust yourself. You are worthy of love, especially your own.

Compassion softened my inner voice. It also reshaped how I approached problems—with less panic, more clarity.

# Strategy Ten: Solving Problems with Clarity and Compassion

*"The problem is not the problem. The problem is your attitude about the problem."*
—**Captain Jack Sparrow** (yes, even pirates can be wise)

## When Emotions Cloud the Path

Caregiving often demands quick decisions in emotionally charged moments. But when we're overwhelmed, it's easy to react rather than respond. I've learned that having a structured approach to problem solving helps me slow down, breathe, and make thoughtful choices that honor both Daryl's needs and my own.

## Steps to Solve Problems Effectively

1. Recognize your discomfort. Emotional distress is often the first signal that something needs attention.

2. Identify the cause. Ask, "Why am I feeling this way?"

Feelings aren't the problem—they point to it.

3. Define the problem. Clarify what's actually creating the discomfort.

4. Brainstorm possible solutions. Let ideas flow freely without judgment.

5. Examine pros and cons. Consider feasibility, effectiveness, and emotional impact.

6. Choose a solution and create an action plan. Map out steps toward resolution.

7. Implement the plan. Put the solution into motion and observe.

8. Evaluate its effectiveness. Was it successful? If not, what got in the way? Adjust and try again.

## A Personal Reframe: Planning for Respite

One morning, sunlight streamed through the blinds as I sat at the kitchen table, a knot tightening in my stomach. Daryl's stiffness was worsening. His voice had become a whisper, and he coughed while eating—each sound triggering my concern. I was preparing to visit my daughter in California for two weeks, and the question loomed: "How can I ensure Daryl's safety while I'm away?"

Daryl insisted he could manage alone. But I knew we

needed a plan. At his next care team meeting, I voiced my concerns. Together, we explored three options:

1. Stay with family
2. Stay in a Transitional Care Unit (TCU)
3. Remain home with support

Options 1 and 2 offered safety and supervision—but Daryl resisted. He wanted to stay in his home, surrounded by familiar routines. So we chose Option 3 and built a detailed action plan:

## Action Plan Highlights

- Activated Honor Alert fall detection
- Occupational Therapist taught fall-prevention techniques
- Physical Therapist focused on strength and balance
- Speech Pathologist addressed voice and swallowing issues
- Social Worker approved 10 hours/week of respite care
- Scheduled transportation to and from his workout
- Increased caregiver hours
- Installed a camera (with Daryl's permission) for safety
- Set up Google Nest for doorbell communication
- Taught Daryl how to microwave freezer meals

This plan gave me peace of mind—and has become our go-to strategy whenever I travel. Each time, I revisit the options and adjust based on Daryl's evolving needs.

## Why It Matters

*Problem solving isn't just about logistics—it's about emotional clarity. A structured approach can:*

- Improve critical thinking
- Build self-confidence
- Lead to compassionate decisions
- Strengthen relationships

## Tools That Help

- **Reframe the problem:** Shift your perspective to uncover new solutions
- **Break it down:** Tackle one piece at a time
- **Stay positive:** Believe a solution is possible
- **Involve the care team:** Their insights are invaluable
- **Digital calendars:** Keep everyone informed and aligned
- **Wearable devices:** Add a layer of safety
- **Communication platforms:** Weekly Zoom calls keep our family connected

# Closing Reflection

Solving problems thoughtfully has allowed me to take needed respite without guilt. It's a skill that brings clarity to chaos—and compassion to caregiving. Some problems couldn't be solved in the moment. But they could be written through.

# Strategy Eleven: Journaling—Writing Through the Storm

*"Journal writing is a voyage to the interior."*
**—Christina Baldwin**

## What Is Journaling?

Journaling is the practice of regularly writing down thoughts, feelings, experiences, and reflections. It is a flexible tool that can be a safe place for free expression, problem solving, and documenting personal growth.

While people have kept journals for centuries, psychologist Dr. James Pennebaker helped bring journaling into the realm of emotional healing. His research showed that expressive writing can improve mental and physical health by helping us process trauma, reduce stress, and gain clarity. For caregivers, journaling can be a quiet refuge—a place to sort through the chaos and reconnect with your inner voice.

# A Personal Reframe

One evening, after a long day of appointments and medication adjustments, I sat down with a cup of hot chocolate and opened my journal. I didn't know what I needed to say—I just knew I needed to say something. I wrote about Daryl's quiet strength, my exhaustion, and the moment he smiled at me when I helped him into bed. That smile reminded me why I keep showing up.

Later, I reread that entry and realized: I had captured a moment of grace. Journaling didn't change the circumstances, but it changed how I carried them.

# Why Journaling Matters for Caregivers

Caregiving often pulls you into a cycle of doing—responding, managing, solving. Journaling invites you to pause and reflect. It's a private space where you can name your feelings, explore your fears, celebrate small victories, and even speak to God in the quiet of the page.

- **Reduce stress** by releasing emotional tension
- **Clarify thoughts** when decisions feel overwhelming
- **Track changes** in your loved one's condition or your own reactions
- **Preserve memories** that might otherwise be lost in the rush
- **Reconnect** with yourself beyond your caregiving role

# Tools That Help

- **Prompted journals**: Use questions like "What am I feeling today?" or "What gave me hope?"
- **Voice-to-text apps**: For days when writing feels too hard
- **Gratitude lists**: A simple way to shift perspective
- **Prayer journaling**: Combine reflection with spiritual connection
- **Creative journaling**: Add sketches, quotes, or photos to deepen the experience

# Closing Reflection

Journaling is not about being a writer—it's about being a witness to your own journey. In the pages of your journal, you can be honest, raw, hopeful, and whole. It's a quiet companion that listens without judgment and reminds you that your story matters.

# Getting Started: A Gentle Invitation to Reflect

If you're new to journaling—or simply unsure where to begin—know that there's no right or wrong way to write.

Your journal is a private space, a quiet companion that listens without judgment. Whether you scribble a few lines in a notebook, type into a digital app, or speak your thoughts aloud using voice-to-text, the goal is the same: to give your inner world a place to breathe.

These prompts are designed to meet you where you are. Use them when you feel overwhelmed, grateful, confused, or simply in need of clarity. Let them guide you toward deeper understanding, emotional release, and spiritual renewal.

# Journal Prompts for the Caregiver's Soul

Emotional Check-In

- What emotions have been most present for me today?
- When did I feel most overwhelmed, and what helped me through it?
- What moment today made me feel seen, heard, or appreciated?

Connection & Relationship

- What is one thing I admire about my loved one today?
- How has our relationship changed since I became a caregiver?
- What do I wish I could say to someone who truly understands this journey?

### Faith & Spiritual Grounding

- Where did I feel God's presence today?
- What scripture or prayer is speaking to me right now?
- How has my faith been challenged or strengthened through caregiving?

### Problem Solving & Resilience

- What challenge am I facing right now, and what are three possible ways to approach it?
- What past problem did I solve that I'm proud of? What did I learn from it?
- What resources or people can I lean on this week?

### Hope & Gratitude

- What small joy did I experience today?
- What am I grateful for in this season of life?
- What gives me hope, even on the hardest days?

# Reflection: A Place to Return To

Caregiving can feel like a long, winding road—filled with moments of tenderness, exhaustion, uncertainty, and grace. Journaling offers a quiet place to return to, again and again. It doesn't ask for perfection. It simply invites you to show up as you are.And sometimes, even writing wasn't enough. Sometimes, I just needed to step away.

# Strategy Twelve: Respite—The Gift of Stepping Away

*"You can't pour from an empty cup. Take care of yourself first."*
**—Author Unknown**

## What Is Respite?

Respite care allows you to take a break from caregiving while ensuring your loved one's needs are still met. These breaks can last from a few hours to a few weeks and are essential for maintaining your physical, emotional, and spiritual well-being.

## A Personal Reframe

One of the most powerful examples of respite I've witnessed came from my best friend. Her husband was in hospice, actively dying, and the Memory Care facility couldn't provide the support he needed. She was exhausted—physically and emotionally—and desperately needed rest.

Daryl and I stepped in. We had known their family for years, and Daryl was comfortable with him. Together, we sat by his bedside, held his hand, shared memories, and kept him safe. It was a sacred exchange of care.

If your loved one is capable of joining you in supporting another caregiver, consider bartering time with a trusted friend or couple. It might sound like this:

*"We'll come from 2:00–4:00 p.m. Thursday so you can rest, and it will be great for you to visit for two hours on Friday while I run errands."*

Respite doesn't always mean stepping away alone—it can mean stepping into community.

## Why Respite Matters

*Stepping away from caregiving responsibilities helps you:*

- Rest and recharge
- Exercise or care for your health
- Engage in hobbies
- Run errands or attend appointments
- Be social with friends and family
- Take a trip or simply breathe

Respite isn't selfish—it's strategic. It allows you to return with renewed energy and compassion.

# Tools That Help

- Schedule regular breaks—don't wait until burnout
- Trade time with other caregivers
- Join support groups—online or in-person
- Contact your Area Agency on Aging for services
- Communicate with friends and family for help
- Educate yourself on the value of respite
- Inform respite providers about routines and preferences
- Discuss respite with your loved one to ease guilt or resistance

# Ways to Make It Easier to Take a Break

- **Accept guilt as normal**—but don't let it stop you.
- **Don't ask for permission**—make the decision based on safety and need.
- **Start before you're desperate**—early planning makes transitions smoother.
- **Combine paid services**—with help from others.
- **Frame the caregiver**—as a helper, not a sitter.
- **Check in early**—return a few minutes ahead to observe and reassure, if needed.

# Closing Reflection

It may have been a long time since you've done something just for yourself—even something small like a walk, a warm bath, or a quiet moment with a book. These little things matter. They remind you that you are more than a caregiver—you are a whole person with needs, dreams, and a spirit that deserves rest.

Respite gives you time back. Time to breathe, to heal, to feel like *you* again. Use it before you "need" it. The earlier in your caregiving journey you embrace it, the more sustainable—and joyful—your care will be.

# Affirmation for the Weary Caregiver

*I am worthy of rest.*
*Taking time for myself is not selfish—it is sacred.*
*When I pause to breathe, I renew my strength.*
*When I step away, I do so with love, not guilt.*
*I trust that my loved one is cared for, and I trust that I am*
*allowed to be cared for too.*
*I honor my limits, knowing that doing so allows me to*
*show up with compassion and clarity.*
*I am not alone. I am supported. I am held.*
***Respite is not a retreat—it is a return to myself.***

# The Caregiver's Toolbox: Strategies That Sustain

*Here's a visual summary of the twelve strategies I return to most often. These aren't abstract ideas—they're lived practices, shaped by trial and error and the wisdom of others. Each one offers a way to reset, reconnect, and restore balance—a rhythm of grace that helps me navigate caregiving with clarity and resilience.*

| Strategy | Focus | What It Offers |
|---|---|---|
| Getting Rid of ANTs | Reframing negative thoughts | Emotional clarity, reduced stress |
| Breathing Through the Storm | Mindful breathing | Physical calm, emotional reset |
| The Art of Noticing | Everyday mindfulness | Sensory grounding, presence, resilience |
| Setting Boundaries Without Guilt | Protecting time and energy | Prevent burnout, clarify limits |

| Strategy | Focus | What It Offers |
|---|---|---|
| Let Them Be, Let Yourself Breathe | Releasing control | Emotional freedom, reduced anxiety |
| Rituals That Restore Me | Intentional self-care | Joy, nervous system support, spiritual ease |
| Speak from the "I" | Clear, honest communication | Conflict reduction, self-advocacy |
| From Wishful Thinking to Purposeful Action | Setting SMART goals | Motivation, structure, measurable progress |
| Compassion for the Caregiver | Practicing self-forgiveness | Inner peace, resilience, freedom from guilt |
| Solving Problems with Clarity & Compassion | Step-by-step caregiving decisions | Calm thinking, sustainable solutions |
| Journaling — Writing Through the Storm | Reflective writing | Emotional release, insight, memory keeping |
| Respite — The Gift of Stepping Away | Intentional breaks | Renewal, perspective, caregiver sustainability |

*These strategies aren't just ideas on a page—they're invitations to pause, reset, and choose grace over grit. You don't have to master them all at once. Just begin with one. Let it guide you through the next hard moment, and trust that each small shift is part of a larger healing. You are not alone on this journey—and you are stronger than you know.*

# Expanding the Toolbox—A Personal Reflection

These strategies are not fixed—they've grown with me. What began as survival tactics slowly transformed into rituals of renewal, shaped by trial and error, spiritual anchoring, and the quiet wisdom of others walking this path. As I practiced and refined the twelve core tools in my caregiver toolbox, I found myself yearning for deeper integration—not just coping, but evolving. The following reflection explores how these strategies expanded through structured learning, intuitive listening, and the ongoing dance between resilience and grace.

## A Turning Point: The UCSD Dementia Study

*How structured support helped me build resilience and emotional regulation.*

Caregiving often stirs up feelings of guilt, inadequacy, and anxiety—emotions that can spiral into negative thought patterns. Before participating in the UCSD Dementia Study, I didn't realize that I could change my thinking. When those thoughts escalated, I felt like I was digging myself into a hole. My faith offered comfort and reminded me to surrender what I couldn't control to God. But even in prayer, I sensed I needed more—tools to help me cope. I prayed for guidance, and the opportunity to join the study felt like an answer.

## How the Strategies Evolved

My participation in the UCSD Dementia Study marked a turning point. The study, which began over 40 years ago, demonstrated that cognitive-behavioral interventions could reduce caregiver distress. Dr. Mausbach and his team believed caregivers could learn specific skills to improve mood and overall well-being. The program offered counseling, coping strategies, and access to UCSD's internet-based caregiver platform.

For 15 months, I engaged with the web-based program, including six months of intensive training and follow-ups every six months for two years. Each week, I selected a goal tailored to my caregiving schedule—deciding how often and how long I would engage in the activity. I tracked my progress nightly using an app, rating my mood with one to five hearts.

Weekly 60-minute phone calls with my therapist provided empathetic support and accountability. I took my blood pressure before each session, helping the study analyze how chronic stress affects heart health. The findings were sobering: elevated stress can increase heart rate and blood pressure, contributing to heart disease and stroke.

Every six months, I completed a mood questionnaire. Over time, I discovered which strategies helped stabilize my emotions, strengthen my coping skills, and improve my overall well-being.

## Strategies I Learned:

- Getting rid of ANTs (Automatic Negative Thoughts)
- Deep breathing
- Mindfulness
- Setting boundaries without guilt
- Stress relief rituals
- "I" messages
- SMART goals
- Self-compassion

Participating in the study was truly life-changing.

# Reinforcement and Growth: APDA's Virtual Caregiver Class

*Building on foundational tools with new techniques and peer support.*

After the study, I sought new ways to reinforce and

expand what I'd learned. I enrolled in a six-week virtual caregiver class offered by APDA's Northwest Chapter.

Our resource was *The Caregiver Helpbook*, which introduced practical tools for:

- **Reducing stress** through exercise, relaxation, and medical check-ups
- **Managing emotions** like guilt, anger, and depression
- **Building confidence** in handling caregiving demands
- **Managing time**, setting goals, and solving problems
- **Communicating feelings** effectively
- **Making tough decisions**
- **Locating helpful resources**

Following the course, I joined a support group of past participants. Each month, we set and shared SMART goals, reflected on our progress, and learned from guest speakers specializing in Parkinson's and caregiving. These sessions deepened our learning and held us accountable.

# A New Philosophy: "Let Them, Let Me"

*Learning to release control and reclaim peace through intentional response.*

During a visit to my daughter in San Luis Obispo, we hiked through Montana de Oro State Park. Afterward, we settled into beach chairs overlooking the cliffs, sharing thoughts under whispering breezes and golden sun. Cheri introduced me to a philosophy she'd adopted: "Let Them." Inspired by Mel Robbins, it's about releasing the need to control others and allowing them to be who they are.

That idea stayed with me. I bought Robbins' book—one for myself and one for a friend recovering from surgery—and began listening to her podcasts and reading her emails. I started applying "Let Them" in caregiving and beyond.

But as I turned the pages, I realized what I'd been missing: the "Let Me." What do I choose after letting go? That's the part that requires intention.

For example, when Daryl resists wearing his hearing aids, I "let him" make his own choices. Our son created a workaround by routing TV sound through the aids, and Daryl discovered he could mute the sound with just one. I "let him" and trust the audiologist will address it at his next appointment. Meanwhile, the "Let Me" allows me to focus on gratitude—that the violent sounds no longer fill our apartment, and I can hear birdsong again as I write in my journal.

*"Healing yourself can be messy. It may hurt at first, but it is ultimately for your highest good. The dark clouds of rainfall are necessary for new growth."*
**—Yung Pueblo**

## Strategy in Practice: What I Use Most

*Letting go, leaning in, and living with intention.*

"Let Them" comes naturally. It helps me release what I

can't control and focus on what I can—my reactions. "Let Me" is a work in progress. It shows up in small moments: taking deep breaths, sipping hot chocolate as I journal, closing my eyes in gratitude for our simple, sufficient home, or walking in nature—my ritual of renewal.

When I need to start a new strategy or refine one I haven't yet internalized, I turn to SMART goals. They give structure to my growth.

# Looking Back: What I Would Tell My Younger Self

*It's never too late to begin.*

These strategies are a lifelong practice. I wish I had learned them earlier—as a child, a wife, a mother, a friend, a teacher. They're not just for caregivers; they're for anyone seeking emotional resilience and peace.

Start with one. Set it as a SMART goal. Evaluate your progress daily or weekly. Give yourself grace. It takes intentional work.

Over time, I realized that even the best strategies couldn't carry me through every storm. There were moments when the checklist faded, when coping tools felt distant, and all that remained was the ache. In those spaces, I stopped striving and started listening—to silence, to memory, to something greater. That's where grace found me.

# PART III

# ANCHORED IN GRACE—REFLECTIONS FROM THE CAREGIVER'S SOUL

*"Grace meets us where we are, not where we pretend to be."*
**—Barbara Brown Taylor**

# When I Am Overwhelmed

The hallway outside the clinic was quiet, but inside me, everything was loud. I clutched the crumpled printout from the doctor's office—words that didn't feel right, a diagnosis that didn't match what I saw in Daryl's eyes, in his movements, in the way he struggled to find words. Something was missing. Something was wrong.

Daryl sat beside me, his hand resting in mine, his gaze distant. I wanted to be strong for him, but my thoughts were spiraling. What if this isn't the right diagnosis? What if we're wasting time? What if things get worse before anyone listens? The weight of the unknown pressed down on me, and I felt myself slipping into fear—grief for a future I couldn't yet name.

I stepped outside into the cold air, trying to breathe. The sky was overcast, the wind sharp. I leaned against the brick wall and whispered the only words I could remember:

*"Therefore do not worry about tomorrow, for tomorrow will worry about itself. Each day has enough trouble of its own."*
**—Matthew 6:34**

The verse didn't erase the fear, but it gave me a foothold. A place to stand. I didn't have to solve tomorrow. I only had to show up for today.

Later that night, I wrote in my journal:

*"Sometimes the bravest thing we do is simply stay present in the storm."*
**—Brené Brown**

And that became my prayer. Not for answers, but for presence. For grace in the waiting. For trust that God was already holding the pieces I couldn't yet see.

# When I Am Afraid

The sun had just dipped below the horizon, casting a soft amber glow across the living room walls. Daryl was in his favorite chair, quiet, his hands resting gently in his lap. I sat across from him, the silence between us filled with the weight of what we now knew: Parkinson's. A disease with no cure. A future we hadn't planned for.

I watched him, trying to memorize the way his eyes still sparkled when he looked at me, even as his body betrayed him. My heart ached with the thought that one day, I might be sitting in this room alone. The fear crept in slowly—like dusk settling over the day—quiet but undeniable.

I stood and walked to the window, pressing my hand against the cool glass. Outside, the world kept moving. Inside, mine felt paused. I whispered a prayer, not for answers, but for courage. And then I remembered the verse that had carried me through so many uncertain moments:

*"Do not fear: I am with you; do not be anxious: I am your God. I will strengthen you, I will help you, I will uphold you with my victorious right hand."*
**—Isaiah 41:10**

The words didn't erase the fear, but they softened it. They reminded me that I wasn't walking this road alone.

Later, I came across a quote that felt like a calm to my soul:

*"Fear never builds the future, but faith does."*
**—Elisabeth Elliot**

So I chose faith. Not because I wasn't afraid, but because I knew that even in the darkest moments, God was already there—holding us both.

# When I Am Worried

I remember standing in the kitchen, the late afternoon light slanting through the window, casting long shadows across the tile floor. Daryl had just gone down for a nap, and the silence in the house felt heavier than usual. The diagnosis was still fresh—Parkinson's. A word that had suddenly reshaped everything.

I stared at the calendar pinned to the fridge, filled with birthdays, appointments, and penciled-in plans for a family trip we'd hoped to take. Ten of us, all together. Would that still be possible? Would Daryl be able to travel? Would we even be able to stay in this house—the one he loved, the one he hoped to live in until the end?

The questions came like waves, each one pulling me further from shore. I gripped the edge of the counter and whispered, "God, I don't know how to do this."

And then, like a thread pulling me back to center, I remembered the verse:

*"It is the Lord who goes before you; he will be with you and will never fail you or forsake you. So do not fear or be dismayed."*
**—Deuteronomy 31:8**

I closed my eyes and let the words settle. I didn't need to have all the answers. I didn't need to map out the future. I only needed to trust that God was already there—walking ahead, clearing the path, holding us steady.

Later that evening, I came across a quote that felt like it had been written just for me:

*"Worry does not empty tomorrow of its sorrow, it empties today of its strength."*
—**Corrie ten Boom**

So I chose to breathe. To be present. To believe that even in the uncertainty, we were not alone.

# When I Feel Doubtful

The air was thick with late-summer humidity, and the scent of dry leaves hinted that fall was just around the corner. I sat at the kitchen table, papers spread out before me—blueprints, city correspondence, notes from the architect. Daryl was resting in the next room, and I could hear the soft hum of his breathing, steady but slow.

I stared at the plans again. Two feet. Just two feet across the north side of the garage, and yet it felt like the entire project was unraveling. The city hadn't approved the blueprints. The architect needed to revise them. Time was slipping away, and with each passing day, the dream of our apartment—our sanctuary—felt more distant.

Doubt crept in like a shadow at dusk. I began to question everything. Was God really watching over us? Did He want the best for us? I found myself focusing on the obstacles, the delays, the uncertainty. My heart felt heavy, and my prayers felt hollow.

I walked outside and sat on the porch steps, letting the cool breeze brush against my face. The maple tree across in the neighbor's yard had begun to turn, its leaves tinged with gold. I closed my eyes and whispered, "Lord, I don't understand."

And then, like a gentle nudge, the verse came to mind:

*"Trust in the Lord with all your heart and lean not on your own understanding; in all your ways submit to him, and he will make your paths straight."*
**—Proverbs 3:5-6**

I didn't need to understand. I needed to trust.

Later, I came across a quote that felt like it had been written just for me:

*"Faith is not the absence of doubt, but the means to overcome it."*
**—Steven Furtick**

So I chose to believe—not because the path was clear, but because the One who guides us never loses His way.

# When I'm Feeling Lonely

The wind howls outside the apartment window, rattling the panes like an impatient visitor. Snow piles up in silent drifts along the sill, and the thermometer reads a number so low it feels more like a dare than a temperature. Minnesota in deep winter doesn't just chill the skin—it isolates. The neighborhood streets are deserted, the sky a dull gray, and the world feels paused.

Inside, the apartment is quiet. Too quiet. My loved one sits in his recliner, nestled in his bright green down jacket, his eyes distant. When he speaks, it's barely a whisper—slurred, breathy, like the words are slipping away before they reach me. I lean in, trying to catch them, trying to connect. But the silence between us stretches longer than the sentences he can form. I nod, smile, hold his hand. Still, the loneliness creeps in like the cold seeping through the walls.

I move to the window, watching the snow swirl under the streetlight. I feel the ache of solitude—not just the absence of people, but the absence of conversation, of shared laughter, of being understood. The kind of loneliness that caregiving sometimes brings, when love is present but words are not.

And then I remember.

I close my eyes and breathe in the stillness.

*"God is our refuge and our strength, an ever-present help in distress."*
**—Psalm 46**

The verse from Psalm 46 rises in my heart like a warm ember. I don't need to speak aloud. I don't need to go anywhere. God is here—in the hush of the room, in the quiet companionship of my loved one, in the very breath I take.

I reach out—not with my hands, but with my spirit. And I feel it: a presence that doesn't need words. A comfort that fills the space between us. A reminder that even in the loneliest moments, I am never truly alone.

Later that afternoon, when the wind eased and the sun broke through the clouds in a pale shimmer, I bundled up and stepped outside. The snow crunched beneath my boots, and the air stung my cheeks, but it felt good to move. I walked slowly down the alley behind the garage, past the bare trees and the frozen lake. A crow called out from a branch above, and I paused to listen. The world was still here—alive, breathing, waiting.

I thought of a quote I'd once tucked into my journal, now resurfacing like a gentle nudge:

*"In every walk with nature one receives far more than he seeks."*
**—John Muir**

# When I Feel Stretched and in a Time Crunch

The clock blinked 3:42 p.m. as I stood in the kitchen, reheating a cup of hot chocolate I'd already forgotten twice. My phone buzzed with a text from a friend: "Want to grab a quick walk later?" I stared at it, torn. The laundry wasn't folded. Daryl had a medical appointment in the morning. Dinner still needed prepping. My calendar felt like a puzzle missing half its pieces.

I sighed and set the mug down. The idea of stepping away—even for an hour—felt indulgent. But beneath the guilt was something else: longing. I missed conversations that didn't revolve around medications or symptoms. I missed laughter. I missed being seen.

I walked to the window and watched the breeze stir the leaves. That's when the verse came to mind, like a whisper in the quiet:

*"...not giving up meeting together, as some are in the habit of doing, but encouraging one another—and all the more as you see the Day approaching."*
**—Hebrews 10:25**

I knew the truth: connection wasn't a luxury. It was a lifeline. Other believers had lifted me in prayer, held space for my grief, reminded me that I wasn't walking this road alone. And every time I made space for community, I felt replenished—more present, more grounded, more able to care for Daryl with grace.

Later that evening, I came across a quote that echoed what my heart already knew:

*"Almost everything will work again if you unplug it for a few minutes... including you."*
**—Anne Lamott**

So I texted back: **"Yes. I'd love that walk."** And in that small act of connection, I chose restoration over exhaustion.

# When I Feel Weary

It was late—past midnight—and the apartment was quiet except for the hum of the refrigerator and the occasional creak of the floorboards below. I lay in bed staring at the ceiling, my mind racing through the day's decisions: the downsizing, the move, Daryl's resistance, the logistics of caregiving. I had tried to sleep, but my thoughts kept looping like a broken record. What if this was the wrong choice? What if he never felt at home again?

Earlier that evening, Daryl had looked around the new space with a mix of confusion and sadness. "I just miss our old place," he whispered, his voice barely audible. I nodded, trying to hold back tears. I missed it too—the creaky hardwood floors, the covered patio, the memories etched into every corner. But I also knew we couldn't go back.

That night, I felt bone-tired. Not just physically, but emotionally—like I was carrying a weight I couldn't set down. I reached for my journal, hoping to quiet the noise in my head. Instead, I found myself flipping to a verse I'd scribbled weeks earlier:

*"Come to me, all you who are weary and burdened, and I will give you rest..."*
**—Matthew 11:28**

I didn't feel rested. But I did feel seen. That verse wasn't a magic fix—it didn't erase the exhaustion or the ache of transition. But it reminded me that I wasn't alone in it. That even in the middle of the night, in a new apartment that didn't yet feel like home, I could lean into something larger than myself. I could rest—not in certainty, but in trust.

Caregiving stretches you in ways you never expect. It asks for everything, and then a little more. But in that quiet moment, I let myself exhale. I didn't have all the answers. I didn't need to. I just needed to rest, and remember that I was held.

And maybe, rest itself was part of the healing. I thought of a quote I'd once tucked into the back of my planner, now resurfacing in my mind like a gentle whisper:

*"Rest is not idleness, and to lie sometimes on the grass under trees on a summer's day... is by no means a waste of time."*
**—John Lubbock**

Even in the midst of caregiving, rest could be sacred. Not a pause from purpose, but a quiet affirmation that I was still whole.

# When I Am Disappointed

The sun descended into the horizon, setting the sky ablaze in molten gold and crimson as I sank onto the ship's deck bench. The waves lapped in steady whispers against the hull, and a cool sea breeze tangled in my hair. Pages of my novel fluttered in the wind, but I hadn't turned a single one—my gaze was fixed on that small break in the clouds where shafts of sunlight pierced the dusk.

I lifted my eyes toward the distant curve of Mount Fuji, but instead of snow-capped peaks, I saw Daryl. I remembered him at dinner: fumbling the laminated menu, fingers trembling so badly he spilled his soda. The easy grace with which he once moved—up the gangway, across a crowded promenade—felt as impossible now as reaching that horizon line.

Disappointment rolled over me in waves. This voyage we'd planned together—our dream of adventure and laughter—had become a mirror of what Parkinson's had quietly stolen. Alone on this deck, the ship's hum felt like a pulsing ache in my chest. I closed my eyes, trying to steady the grief for the future we'd imagined but could no longer share.

A verse rose in my mind, soft and familiar:

*"The Lord is close to the broken-hearted and saves those who are crushed in spirit."*
**—Psalm 34:18**

I didn't feel saved. But I felt held, if only by that promise. The sea's steady breath and the fading light reminded me that even in loss, something deeper could carry me through.

I took a slow breath and let a favorite line drift into the stillness:

> *"The wound is the place where the light enters you."*
> **—Rumi**

In that gilded moment, I realized disappointment could be a doorway—not to what I'd lost, but to unexpected healing. The sun slipped behind the clouds, and though the sky darkened, a single ray lingered across the water, and I trusted it would linger in me, too.

# When I Choose Acceptance

*"To have and to hold from this day forward, for better, for worse, for richer, for poorer, in sickness and in health..."*
**—Marriage Vows**
*"Love bears all things, believes all things, hopes all things, endures all things. Love never ends."*
**—I Corinthians 13:7-8**

There came a moment when I stopped resisting Parkinson's—not because I gave up, but because I gave in to grace. Acceptance wasn't a passive surrender. It was an active choice to love Daryl as he is now, not as he was before. I realized he is still the man I chose to marry, still the partner I vowed to cherish in sickness and in health.

When I chose acceptance, I stopped measuring our life by what we'd lost. I began to see what remained—and what could still be created. We couldn't go to A *Christmas Carol* at the Guthrie Theater anymore, but we could invite friends over to play cards. The joy was still there, just in a different form.

Acceptance allowed us to cope as a team. It gave me permission to stop striving for what used to be and start embracing what is. I let go of the past and stepped into the present, where love lives in the everyday:

- Daryl scraping dishes and loading the dishwasher

- Spraying stains, folding laundry, riding the chair lift with groceries
- Getting dressed on his own, asking for help when needed
- Triking around Lake Nokomis, attending church online
- Showing up for grandchildren's events, visiting friends, joining support groups
- Shopping together, managing medications, attending appointments
- Advocating for his needs—with dignity, patience, and love

These small acts preserve his independence and remind us both that he is still capable, still whole, still Daryl.

Acceptance doesn't mean I never feel grief or frustration. It means I choose to anchor myself in love, again and again. And love, when rooted in grace, does not diminish with illness—it deepens.

# Reflections From the Caregiver's Soul

Caregiving is not only a physical and emotional journey—it is a spiritual one. After life unraveled and I leaned on strategies to cope, I found myself returning again and again to the quiet places of the soul. In moments of loneliness, fear, doubt, and exhaustion, I discovered that faith was not just a comfort—it was a lifeline.

Part IV is a collection of reflections born from those

moments. They are not polished answers, but honest prayers—scenes where grace met me in the middle of the mess. My hope is that these words offer you rest, encouragement, and a reminder: you are never walking alone.

# PART IV
# A PAUSE FOR MY SOUL

*"In the midst of movement and chaos, keep stillness inside of you."*
**—Deepak Chopra**

# Sanctuary of Prayer

Prayers for peace, clarity, and strength in the caregiving journey.

As this memoir gently draws to a close, I invite you into a quiet sanctuary—a space to rest, reflect, and reconnect with your soul. Before we turn toward resources and next steps, let these timeless prayers offer you comfort and clarity. Whether you are just beginning your caregiving journey, walking through its most demanding hours, or looking back with tender remembrance, may these words meet you where you are—and remind you that you are never alone.

**The Peace Prayer of St. Francis of Assisi** reminds us that even in our weariness, we can be vessels of peace and love.

### Peace Prayer of St. Francis of Assisi

*Lord, make me an instrument of your peace:*
*where there is hatred, let me sow love;*
*where there is injury, pardon;*
*where there is doubt, faith;*
*where there is despair, hope;*
*where there is darkness, light;*
*where there is sadness, joy.*

*O divine Master, grant that I may not so much seek*
*to be consoled as to console,*
*to be understood as to understand,*
*to be loved as to love.*
*For it is in giving that we receive,*

*it is in pardoning that we are pardoned,*
*and it is in dying that we are born to eternal life.*
**The Serenity Prayer** offers the wisdom to discern what we can carry, and what we must release.

### Serenity Prayer
*God, grant me the serenity to accept the things I cannot change, the courage to change the things I can, and the wisdom to know the difference.*
**—Reinhold Niebuh**

## Prayer for Stillness and Strength

May I find quiet in the noise,
peace in the pressure,
and grace in the grind.
May I breathe deeply when the day feels heavy,
and remember that rest is not weakness,
but wisdom.
May I be gentle with myself,
and open to the help that comes—
in unexpected moments,
from unexpected places.
Let stillness be my sanctuary,
and love my compass
as I walk this sacred path.

Together, they form a quiet benediction—a breath before the next step. This chapter becomes a **spiritual interlude**—a moment of pause before the practical turn.

# Bridging the Inner and Outer Journey

In Parts II, III, and IV, we explored the emotional terrain of caregiving—the self-talk, the reframing, the quiet courage it takes to offer yourself grace in the midst of daily demands. These strategies are the heartbeat of resilience. They help us stay grounded when the ground beneath us shifts.

But inner strength doesn't mean going it alone. Caregiving also requires scaffolding—practical supports that hold us up when our own reserves run low. I learned, often through trial and error, that there are organizations, tools, and communities designed to help. They don't replace the personal work, but they make it more sustainable. They offer clarity when the fog rolls in, and connection when isolation creeps close.

Now, we turn outward. The next section gathers the lifelines that helped me find clarity, connection, and courage. May they do the same for you.

Caregiving is both an inward and outward journey—one that asks us to listen deeply and reach bravely. As we move forward, I invite you to carry the strength you've cultivated and the grace you've claimed. What follows is a gathering of support: organizations, tools, and communities that helped me stay steady when the road grew steep. Let this next section be your companion—a map of possibility and connection. Take a breath. Turn the page when you're ready.

# PART V
# RESOURCES FOR THE JOURNEY

*"The journey of a thousand miles begins with a single step."*
**— Lao Tzu**

*"Caregiving often calls us to lean into love we didn't know possible."*
**— Tia Walker**

# National Organizations and Helplines

When I felt overwhelmed or unsure, these organizations offered clarity, compassion, and practical help. Whether through a phone call, a downloadable guide, or a webinar, they reminded me that we weren't alone—and that support was always within reach.

| Organization | Support Offered | Website | Phone |
|---|---|---|---|
| **American Parkinson Disease Association (APDA)** | Support groups, exercise programs, helpline | www.apdaparkinson.org | 800-223-2732 |
| **Parkinson's Foundation** | Webinars, care helpline | www.parkinson.org | 800-473-4636 |
| **Michael J. Fox Foundation** | Research, clinical trials, care guides | www.michaeljfox.org | 800-708-7644 |

| Organization | Support Offered | Website | Phone |
|---|---|---|---|
| Family Caregiver Alliance (FCA) | Education, legal help, emotional support | www.caregiver.org | 800-445-8106 |
| VA Caregiver Support | Respite, training, peer support | www.caregiver.va.gov | 855-260-3274 |
| Parkinson Canada | Care guides, webinars, podcasts | www.parkinson.ca | 888-664-1974 |
| National Institute on Aging | Aging and health condition info | www.nia.nih.gov | 800-222-2225 |
| Caregiver Coalition of San Diego | Support groups, handbook | www.caregivercoalitionsd.org | 858-505-6435 |

In the midst of caregiving, support can arrive quietly—a voice on the phone, a guide in your inbox, a reminder that you are not alone. These organizations became part of my circle of care, offering strength when mine ran low. As you explore these resources, may you find not just information, but connection. May they help you breathe a little easier, and remind you that help is never far away.

# Tools, Stories, and Support for the Road Ahead

Caregiving is never a solo act—even when it feels like one. In the quiet hours, when exhaustion sets in and answers feel far away, I learned to reach outward. Over time, I discovered organizations, websites, phone numbers, and support networks that helped me feel less alone and more equipped. These lifelines didn't solve every problem, but they offered clarity, connection, and sometimes just the right answer at the right time.

This section gathers those lifelines in one place. They are not exhaustive, but they are meaningful. These are the companions I found along the way—resources that lightened my load and strengthened my heart.

May they help you breathe easier, find answers faster, and feel less alone on the road ahead.

Let's walk forward together—with grace in our hearts and help in our hands.

When the path feels overwhelming, national organizations and helplines can offer clarity, guidance, and a steady voice on the other end of the line. These resources are more than just websites—they're lifelines, especially in moments of uncertainty.

Whether you're seeking medical information, emotional

support, or practical tools, these organizations have helped thousands of families—including ours—navigate the complexities of Parkinson's with greater confidence and connection.

# You Tube Channels and Video Resources

*Sometimes, seeing someone else walk a similar path can be more powerful than words alone. These YouTube channels offer expert advice, personal stories, exercise routines, and emotional support for both people with Parkinson's and their caregivers.*

## Speech & Voice Therapy

- **SPEAK OUT! by Parkinson Voice Project**
  Guided therapy and exercises led by speech-language pathologists.
- **SPEAK OUT! Home Practice Sessions**
  Live sessions held Monday through Friday at 10 A.M. U.S. Central Time.
- **What Is Parkinson's?**
  Overview of Parkinson's disease from the Parkinson Voice Project.

# Exercise & Wellness

- **American Parkinson Disease Association (APDA)**
  Educational videos including *Let's Keep Moving with APDA*.
- **Power for Parkinson's**
  Free exercise classes and wellness content.
- **Parkinson's Foundation**
  Wellness programs for all stages of Parkinson's.
- **The Gut & Parkinson's Connection**
  Hosted by Dr. Gilbert, exploring gut health and Parkinson's.

# Emotional Support & Personal Growth

- **Mel Robbins**
  Videos on mindset, stress relief, and caregiver burnout.
- **Brené Brown**
  Talks on vulnerability, empathy, and self-compassion.
- **Careblazers**
  Self-care strategies and free caregiver resources.
- **Family Caregiver Alliance**
  Personal stories, stress management, self-care, and research.

# Education & Expert Insights

*When I first stepped into the role of caregiver, I didn't know what I didn't know. These resources helped me build a foundation—not just of facts, but of confidence. They offer clear explanations, expert interviews, and wellness strategies that speak to both the science of Parkinson's and the lived experience of those affected by it.*

*Whether you're looking for guidance on symptom management, mental health, or simply how to get through the day with more ease, these trusted sources have helped me feel less alone and more equipped.*

- **Parkinson's Foundation**
  Hundreds of videos on Parkinson's basics, relaxation, and expert interviews.
- **Davis Phinney Foundation**
  Wellness tips and community stories focused on living well today.
- **Parkinson Canada**
  Webinars on symptom management, DBS, sleep, and more.
- **Veterans Health Administration (VA)**
  Videos on Parkinson's, mental health, and caregiver support.

# Personal Stories & Caregiver Perspectives

*Caregiving is not just a role—it's a relationship. These stories reflect the emotional depth, resilience, and shared humanity of those walking the Parkinson's path.*

- **The Secret Life of Parkinson's**
  Created by Jessica Krauser, featuring candid conversations.
- **Stanford APDA Caregiver Playlist**
  Talks by Dave Iverson and Barbara Sheklin Davis.
- **Home Instead Senior Care Resources**
  Tips for caring for senior loved ones.
- **Lianna Marie – Lessons Learned as a Caregiver**
  Reflections and insights from her experience caring for her mother.
- **Not Just "Caregivers", We Are Partners in Parkinson's**
  Larry Gifford and his wife, Rebecca, share their journey of partnership.

# Podcasts and Audio Resources

*Sometimes, the most comforting voice is one that says, "Me too."*
**—Sharon Jaynes**

Whether I'm walking, driving, or simply trying to make sense of the day, podcasts offer connection, education, and companionship. These audio resources helped me feel less alone and more informed.

I discovered Larry Gifford's podcast *When Life Gives You Parkinson's* shortly after Daryl was first diagnosed. I was searching for anything that could help me understand what Parkinson's really meant—not just the clinical definitions, but the lived experience. Larry's voice became a companion on my own journey. He said something in one of the early episodes that stopped me in my tracks:

*"When I was diagnosed with Parkinson's, all our plans went poof. There was no way to plan, had no control. The only thing I could control is ME."*

That resonated deeply. I knew that feeling—the sudden loss of certainty, the scramble to find footing. His honesty helped me name what I was feeling and gave me permission to begin reframing our new reality.

Larry, who was the National Director of Talk Radio, used his platform to amplify voices that often go unheard. His podcast became a lifeline for me—not just for information, but for emotional clarity.

In another podcast, I heard Dr. Ray Dorsey of the Mayo Clinic say:

*"If people with Parkinson's do not start telling their stories, we will never raise enough money to do anything in any way to cure it."*

That was my turning point. I thought, There it is. I'm a storyteller. How can I expect anyone else to share their truth if I'm not willing to share mine? That moment helped shape my own commitment to writing this memoir—not just for Daryl and me, but for others walking this path.

## Featured Podcasts

- **When Life Gives You Parkinson's**
  Hosted by Larry Gifford and supported by Parkinson Canada, this podcast chronicles Larry's personal journey with Parkinson's and features stories from patients, families, care partners, and researchers.
- **Substantial Matters: Life and Science of Parkinson's**
  Produced by the Parkinson's Foundation, this podcast features interviews with medical experts on treatments, symptom management, and emerging research.
- **The Michael J. Fox Foundation Parkinson's Podcast**
  This series explores the latest in Parkinson's research, drug development, and advocacy, alongside personal

stories from patients and caregivers.

# Bonus Resource

- **Expert Briefing Webinars**
  Hour-long webinars from the Parkinson's Foundation covering symptom management and care strategies. Visit www.parkinson.org for upcoming sessions.

# Available On

- Apple Podcasts
- Spotify

# Recommended Books and Guides

*Caregiving for someone with Parkinson's—or any progressive illness—is a journey marked by uncertainty, adaptation, and deep emotional labor. These books have been selected not only for their practical value, but for their ability to speak to the heart of the caregiver experience. Whether you're seeking clinical clarity, emotional validation, or a sense of companionship through memoir, this curated list offers a range of voices and perspectives to support you.*

## Clinical Guidance & Practical Tools

Books that offer expert strategies, treatment insights, and actionable advice for navigating care.

- **The New Parkinson's Disease Treatment Book** by J. *Eric Ahlskog, MD*
  A Mayo Clinic movement specialist empowers patients and caregivers to collaborate with clinicians and explore treatment options.
- **Everything You Need to Know About CAREGIVING for Parkinson's Disease** by *Leanna Marie*
  A comprehensive guide that balances care strategies

with caregiver self-care.

- **Passages in Caregiving: Turning Chaos into Confidence** by *Gail Sheehy*
  Outlines nine critical steps for navigating the caregiving journey with clarity and courage.
- **The Caregiver's Companion** by *Carolyn A. Brent*
  Offers practical advice for handling medical, legal, and emotional challenges in caregiving.
- **You Are a Better Caregiver Than You Think** by *Kevin Klos*
  Practical solutions from a movement disorder specialist and caregiver to his mother.
- **The Caregiver Helpbook**
  Tools to reduce stress, build confidence, set goals, and communicate effectively.
  *Used in my six-week virtual training through APDA Northwest. Easy to read and offers both practical advice and emotional support to help caregivers thrive and find resources during their challenging journey.*

# Emotional Support & Mindset Shifts

These books are more than advice manuals—they are lifelines for emotional survival and growth. They offer caregivers the language, perspective, and validation needed to navigate the inner terrain of caregiving with greater resilience and self-compassion.

- **The Emotional Survival Guide for Caregivers** by *Barry Jacobs*
  Offers psychological insight into managing guilt, stress, and burnout. This book reassured me that feelings of resentment, guilt, and isolation are normal reactions that go with the territory of caregiving.
- **The Let Them Theory** by *Mel Robbins*
  Encourages releasing control over others and focusing on your own peace and responses. This book was transformative to me—clearing a path to self-acceptance and freedom, shifting away from controlling others to controlling my actions and responses. It's a strategy I use daily and included in Part II.
- **Advice From a Parkinson's Wife: 20 Lessons Learned the Hard Way** by *Barbara Sheklin Davis*
  Shares hard-earned wisdom for navigating the emotional toll of Parkinson's caregiving.
- **Creating Moments of Joy** by *Jolene Brackey*
  Especially helpful for dementia-related care, emphasizing presence and connection. This book encouraged me to move beyond the negative symptoms of cognitive decline and find opportunities to bring joy, dignity, and happiness into each day.

## Memoirs & Personal Journeys

Stories that reflect the lived experience of caregiving and

living with Parkinson's, offering companionship and perspective.

- **A Parkinson's Life: And a Caregiver's Roadmap** by *Jolyon Hallows*
  A candid account of caregiving for his wife, with practical strategies and emotional insight.
- **A Son's Journey: From Parkinson's Disease Caregiver to Advocate** by *D. George Matthew Ackerman*
  Explores the emotional and logistical realities of caregiving, with a focus on advocacy and resilience.
- **Lucky Man** by *Michael J. Fox*
  A humorous and poignant reflection on living with Parkinson's as a young man. His honesty and humor in facing early diagnosis helped me feel less alone and more hopeful about the future.
- **Always Looking Up: The Adventures of an Incredible Optimist** by *Michael J. Fox*
  A memoir about reframing adversity as opportunity, told with humor and hope. His positive outlook by focusing on everyday blessings and finding silver linings in his struggles are an inspiration to me.
- **No Time Like the Future** by *Michael J. Fox*
  A deeply personal narrative about facing decline with grace, grit, and humor. His reflections on aging and vulnerability helped me embrace my own limitations with more compassion and courage.

# Support Groups and Online Communities

*Support groups and online communities can be lifelines for caregivers and those living with Parkinson's. Whether in person or virtual, these spaces offer connection, education, and emotional support. Many of these programs helped Daryl and me feel less alone, more informed, and more empowered in our journey.*

- **PRESS Program**
  Designed for those diagnosed with PD within the last five years. This eight-week support group helped Daryl and me feel empowered, in control, and optimistic. It provided emotional support and a safe place to share coping strategies.
- **Smart Patients Parkinson's Community**
  In partnership with APDA, this online forum allows individuals with Parkinson's and their care partners to share experiences, advice, and treatment insights in a safe, supportive environment.
- **APDA Virtual Support Groups**
  I found the APDA Northwest six-week Caregiving Class based on *The Caregiver Helpbook* especially helpful. The monthly support group that followed reminded me I wasn't alone. Guest speakers and Q&A sessions deepened our understanding of Parkinson's and our role as caregivers.

- **PMD Alliance**
  Offers Lunch with Docs® webinars—live, interactive discussions with movement disorder neurologists. Provides a welcoming space to learn, ask questions, and connect.
- **VA Veteran's Centers**
  Daryl and I attend a Parkinson's support group for caregivers and partners on the third Thursday of each month. Each session includes a one-hour expert presentation, followed by Q&A and group discussion led by an Occupational Therapist and Social Worker from the Minneapolis VA Clinic.
  *If your partner is a Veteran, contact your closest Veteran's Clinic for more information. www.va.gov (search "Parkinson's support groups" by location)*
- **SPEAK OUT! Home Practice Sessions**
  Live sessions held Monday–Friday at 10 A.M. Central Time. Improves volume, articulation, breath support, vocal quality, intonation, and facial expression. Daryl used this as a refresher course after moving to Minnesota.
- **PD Health @ Home** | Parkinson's Foundation
  Virtual sessions like "Mindfulness Mondays," "Wellness Wednesdays," and "Fitness Fridays," plus a wealth of educational events.
- **Getting Support** | Parkinson's Foundation
  Find the support you need. To locate a support group in your area, call 1-800-473-4636.
- **Facebook Groups**
  Search keywords like "Parkinson's support group,"

"Young Onset Parkinson's," or "Caregivers for Parkinson's." Use the "Groups" tab to filter and explore.

- **Faith Communities**
Larger congregations may host support groups for caregivers. Don't hesitate to ask your local church or synagogue what's available—they may offer more than you expect.

*If you're unsure where to begin, try just one group or forum. Sometimes a single conversation can open the door to connection, clarity, and hope.*

# Local and Regional Resources

*Caregiving can feel overwhelming, but these trusted organizations offer practical support, emotional guidance, and connection—especially for those navigating care in Minnesota. Whether you're planning a respite trip, setting up a caregiving agreement, or simply looking for local services, these resources helped me personally and may help you too.*

- **Minnesota Area Agencies on Aging**
  Connects you to seven regional agencies across Minnesota. They provided me with information on home-delivered meals when I was planning our family respite trip.
- **Senior Linkage Line** Call 1-800-333-2433
  A free, confidential helpline from the Minnesota Board on Aging. They helped me understand the importance of setting up a caregiving agreement with our son before Daryl and I moved into the apartment above his garage.
- **Area Agencies on Aging (National)**
  Search by state to find nearby programs offering respite care, transportation, home modifications, and caregiver support. I used this link to locate resources in the Minneapolis area.

# Intimacy and Connection: Navigating Sexuality with Parkinson's

*Parkinson's reshaped our intimacy—not by erasing it, but by deepening it.*
**—Author Unknown**

**Clinical Overview:**

Motor symptoms, non-motor symptoms, and medication side effects can all impact intimacy.

**Helpful Resources:**

- **ParkinSex Video, Booklet & Kit**
  An experiential guide to intimacy for people with Parkinson's and their partners, developed by APDA with input from clinical sexologist Dr. Sheila Silver.
- **Dr. Regina Koepp's Interview with Dr. Gilbert**
  Available via the Parkinson's Foundation podcast.
- **Intimacy and Parkinson's with Daniel Fleshner and Lisa Thomas**
  Available via Davis Phinney: Foundation for Parkinson's
- **Booklet addresses Relationships, Sex and Parkinson's**
  Available from Parkinson's Organization, UK
- **World Parkinson's Congress Blog**

Gila Bronner's insights on Personal Intimacy and
Sexuality in Parkinson's Disease

**Encouragement to Explore:**

Intimacy may look different—but it can still be beautiful,
affirming, and deeply connective.

# Tools and Apps

*These tools don't replace the hard work of caregiving—but they lighten the load.*

- **Empaira** – A comprehensive caregiving app that supports me with both the emotional and practical sides of care.  It includes:
  - **Community:**  A space where caregivers share feelings, experiences, and encouragement.
  - **Support:**  Emotional check-ins, quick "Reset" exercises for moments of overwhelm, local respite resources, and a library of articles.
  - **Care:**  Tools for appointments, medications, care-team coordination, health tracking, and a customizable Care Card.
- **CareZone** – Medication tracking and shared care notes
- **Find My Friends** – Location tracking in case of wandering
- **Medisafe** – Pill reminders
- **Insight Timer: Meditate and Sleep** – My preferred app for guided meditation. Free, user-friendly, and helpful for stress and anxiety management. I use it nightly to quiet my mind before bed.
- **Aqara Home** – Smart home hub for cameras, locks, lighting, and sensors
- **Google Home/Google Keep** – Front door camera, reminders, voice assistance

- **Aladdin Connect** – Remote garage door access

These tools helped me stay organized and responsive day-to-day. But caregiving isn't just about logistics—it's also about learning, adapting, and finding meaning in the journey.

# Research and Reflection

*Participating in research has helped me deepen my understanding of caregiving and connect with others seeking better ways to cope.*

**Featured Study:**

- **UCSD Caregiver Study**
  An internet-based program teaching coping skills designed to reduce stress and improve emotional well-being. Call 1-858-534-9479

**Impactful Articles & Studies:**

- Rosenberg, E., & Gouge, N. (Age in Action, 22(2))
  *Powerful Tools for Caregivers: Teaching skills that reduce stress and increase self-confidence*
  This article helped me increase self-confidence and reduce stress through SMART goals.
- Kim, D., Peterson, N., & Lee, J. E. (2022)
  *Caregiving outcomes of sub/urban and rural caregivers: The Powerful Tools for Caregivers program. Clinical Gerontologist 1–12*
- Serwe, K.M., & Walmsley, A.L.E. (2021)
  *The effectiveness of telehealth for a caregiver wellness program. Journal of Telemedicine and Telecare, 29(7)*
- Rosney, D.M., Noe, M.F., & Horvath, P.J. (2017)
  *Powerful Tools for Caregivers, a group*

*psychoeducational skill-building intervention for family caregivers. Journal of Caring Sciences, 6(3), 187–198*

**Personal Reflection of SMART Goals:**

Setting SMART goals helped me reclaim time for journaling, track emotional patterns, and deepen my healing.

*One example:*

This week I will record my feelings, an experience, and/ or reflections for twenty minutes before going to bed, three times a week (Monday, Wednesday, and Friday). On Sunday evening, I will evaluate my progress toward my goal.

# Reflections for the Road

These articles helped me reframe my role—not just as a caregiver, but as a learner and advocate.
And yet, beyond the tools and studies, what remains is something quieter and deeper:
The truth that caregiving is a relationship.
One that asks for presence, compassion, and grace—
Not just in the hard moments, but in the ordinary ones, too.
*What follows is a reflection—an offering to every caregiver who has felt unseen, overwhelmed, or quietly strong.*
*To those who carry the weight with tenderness, and walk forward without applause:*
**You are not alone.**

# From My Heart to Yours

*"There are four kinds of people in the world: Those who have been caregivers, those who are currently caregivers, those who will be caregivers,*
*and those who will need caregivers."*
**—Former First Lady Rosalynn Carter**

I believe there's a fifth: those who don't yet realize they've begun the caregiver journey. Their ranks grow daily.

If you're reading this, you may already be one of them. And if so—welcome. These resources are here to guide, support, and remind you that caregiving is not just a role—it's a relationship. One that deserves every ounce of compassion, clarity, and care.

This reflection echoes the themes of my memoir: grief and grace, resilience and renewal, the quiet power of presence. Whether you're just beginning or deep in the journey, may you find strength in your story and peace in your path.

If you're weary, know that you're not weak. You're walking a sacred path—one that asks much, but also gives back in quiet, unexpected ways.

Caregiving taught me that love isn't just what we feel—it's what we choose, again and again, in the quiet moments no one sees.

**Keep going. You're not alone.**

# Reflection

**"When I was weak,
she gave me her strength."**
**—Jimmy Carter**

There are moments in caregiving when strength doesn't
roar—it whispers.
It shows up in quiet gestures, in the willingness to stay, in
the courage to soften.
As the roles shift and the path bends, we learn that love is
not just what we give, but what we allow ourselves to receive.
This reflection is for every care-partner who has felt the
weight of that exchange—and the grace within it.

# Acknowledgements

This memoir would not exist without the love, insight, and support of many people who walked beside me—sometimes quietly, sometimes boldly, always with grace.

To my husband, **Daryl**—thank you for living this story with me. Your courage and tenderness are woven into every page.

To **Brian and Kari**—for your generosity, your vision, and the gift of shared life in our accessible apartment. You made space not just for our bodies, but for our hearts.

To my dear friend, **Trudi**—your friendship has been a lifeline. Your wisdom, humor, and unwavering belief in me gave this story its wings.

To my daughter, **Cheri**—your home in California became my place of respite, renewal, and reflection. Your gentle encouragement helped me embrace the "Let Them" mindset and release what I cannot control. Thank you for reminding me that peace is a place we can choose.

To the caregivers, researchers, and support groups who offered tools, language, and community—especially the **UCSD Caregiver Study**, **Powerful Tools for Caregivers**, and the **Veteran's Support Group hosted by the Minneapolis VA Clinic**, with heartfelt thanks to the presenters from both **Minneapolis** and **Los Angeles**. Your insights helped me find clarity in the chaos.

To the authors, podcasters, and creators whose voices echoed my own experience and helped me feel less alone—thank you for lighting the way.

To the skilled and compassionate professionals at the **Minneapolis VA's Parkinson's and Movement Disorders Program**, your comprehensive care and innovative treatments provided hope and a path forward. I am forever grateful for the support you gave Daryl and me. Thank you to **Rachel**, his occupational therapist, for her wisdom and kindness throughout his journey.

To the authors, podcasters, and creators whose voices echoed my own experience and helped me feel less alone—thank you for lighting the way.

To **Dennis and Derek**— who, with a keen eye for detail, provided invaluable feedback on the manuscript and helped shape my narrative.

To those who have helped—and will help—with editing, publishing, and sharing this story: your care and craft make this work possible. I'm grateful for your partnership in bringing these words into the world.

And to every caregiver walking this path—may you find strength in your story and peace in your path.

# Author's Note

## *Illuminated by grace*

This memoir began as a journal, a quiet place to hold the weight of caregiving and the light that still found its way in. Over time, it became a map—of grief and grace, of resilience and renewal, of the sacred ordinary moments that define a life shared.

If you are a caregiver, know this: your story matters. Your exhaustion does not erase your strength. Your doubts do not diminish your love. You are not invisible.

I wrote this to honor our journey, and to offer companionship to yours. May these pages remind you that caregiving is not just a role—it's a relationship. One built on presence, adaptation, and the kind of love that chooses again and again.

Thank you for reading. Thank you for caring.

*"Only when we are brave enough to explore the darkness will we discover the infinite power of our light."*
**—Brené Brown**

May you feel equipped, even when you feel undone.
May you find grace in the giving, and peace in the path.

# Discussion Questions

This memoir was written not just to share a story, but to spark conversation—about caregiving, illness, resilience, and love. Whether you're reading alone, with a book group, or among fellow caregivers, these questions are offered as a way to reflect, connect, and explore your own journey alongside mine.

## Understanding Caregiving and Parkinson's

- How did this memoir shift your understanding of what it means to be a caregiver or live with a progressive illness like Parkinson's?
- What details or descriptions of Parkinson's—both motor and non-motor symptoms—stood out to you? Were any particularly surprising or eye-opening?
- How did the memoir explore what it means to live with the disease, beyond managing symptoms?

## Personal Connection and Emotional Impact

- Which chapter or anecdote resonated most deeply

with you, and why?

- Did the author's writing style help you connect emotionally to her experience? In what ways did you relate to her story?
- The memoir describes the shift from spouse to caregiver. What were your thoughts on this transition? How does it reflect or differ from your own experience?

## Coping Strategies and Support

- How did the caregiver navigate both the practical and emotional challenges of her role?
- Emotions like frustration, guilt, and loneliness were openly explored. Did any of the coping strategies she used feel helpful or familiar to you?
- Part Two offered a toolbox of strategies. Which one felt most useful or applicable to your own caregiving journey?
- Part Four highlighted several resources. Was there one that you found especially helpful or that you'd like to explore further?

## Reflection and Meaning

- In what ways did Parkinson's affect family relationships

in the memoir? Did anything mirror your own family dynamics?

- Quotes were woven throughout the book. Which one stayed with you, and why?

# Resources Appendix

*Note for print readers*: Web links mentioned throughout the book are listed here in the Resources Appendix for easy reference.

## Part V – Professional Organizations and Helplines

*These trusted organizations offer education, support, and helplines for caregivers and those living with Parkinson's. Many provide webinars, local programs, and expert guidance.*

APDA

- **Support:** Support groups, exercise programs, helpline
- **Website:** apdaparkinson.org
- **Phone:** 800-223-2732

Parkinson's Foundation

- **Support:** Webinars, expert care, nurse helpline
- **Website:** parkinson.org
- **Phone:** 800-473-4636

Michael J. Fox Foundation

- **Support:** Research, clinical trials, care guides
- **Website:** michaeljfox.org
- **Phone:** 800-708-7644

## Family Caregiver Alliance

- **Support:** Education, legal help, emotional support
- **Website:** caregiver.org
- **Phone:** 800-445-8106

## VA Caregiver Support

- **Support:** Respite, training, peer support
- **Website:** caregiver.va.gov
- **Phone:** 855-260-3274

## Parkinson Canada

- **Support:** Care guides, webinars, podcasts
- **Website:** parkinson.ca
- **Phone:** 888-664-1974

## National Institute on Aging

- **Support:** Aging and health condition info
- **Website:** nia.nih.gov
- **Phone:** 800-222-2225

## Caregiver Coalition of San Diego

- **Support:** Support groups, free handbook

- **Website:** caregivercoalitionsd.org
- **Phone:** 858-505-643

# Part V – YouTube Channels and Video Resources

*These YouTube channels and video playlists offer education, personal stories, and caregiver support. They're great for visual learners and those seeking real-life perspectives.*
The Secret Life of Parkinson's

- **Focus:** Personal stories and lived experience
- **Link:** youtube.com/@thesecretlifeofparkinsons

Stanford APDA Playlist

- **Focus:** Caregiver talks and expert interviews
- **Link:** Stanford APDA Playlist

Partners in Parkinson's

- **Focus:** Larry & Rebecca Gifford's story
- **Link:** youtube.com/watch?v=p-6LzqWO8UQ

Mel Robbins

- **Focus:** Mindset and caregiver burnout
- **Link:** youtube.com/@melrobbins

## Careblazers

- **Focus:** Caregiver self-care strategies
- **Link:** careblazers.com

## Davis Phinney Foundation

- **Focus:** Living well with Parkinson's
- **Link:** davisphinneyfoundation.org

## VA Health Videos

- **Focus:** PD and mental health
- **Link:** caregiver.va.gov

## Home Instead Resources

- **Focus:** Senior caregiving tips
- **Link:** homeinstead.com/care-resources

## Lianna Marie – Lessons Learned

- **Focus:** Caregiver reflections
- **Link:** youtube.com/watch?v=cQjeL664woM

# Part V – Podcasts and Audio Resources

*These podcasts offer expert interviews, personal stories, and practical advice for caregivers and those living with Parkinson's.*

When Life Gives You Parkinson's

- **Focus:** Hosted by Larry Gifford; personal stories and interviews
- **Link:** youtube.com/watch?v=-GwJ_uNYyKY

Substantial Matters

- **Focus:** Expert interviews and research from Parkinson's Foundation
- **Link:** parkinson.org/podcast

Michael J. Fox Foundation Podcast

- **Focus:** Research, advocacy, and caregiver stories
- **Link:** michaeljfox.org/podcast

Expert Briefing Webinars

- **Focus:** Symptom management and care strategies
- **Link:** parkinson.org

**Available On:** Apple Podcasts, Spotify, YouTube

# Part V – Support Groups and Online Communities

*These support groups and online communities offer connection, education, and emotional support for caregivers and people with Parkinson's.*

## PRESS Program

- **Focus:** Support group for newly diagnosed individuals
- **Link:** apdaparkinson.org

## Smart Patients Parkinson's Community

- **Focus:** Online forum for sharing experiences and treatment insights
- **Link:** smartpatients.com

## APDA Virtual Support Groups

- **Focus:** Caregiving classes and monthly support groups
- **Link:** apdaparkinson.org

## PMD Alliance

- **Focus:** Webinars and neurologist Q&A
- **Link:** pmdalliance.org

## Lunch with Docs®

- **Focus:** Interactive webinar series from PMD Alliance

- **Link:** pmdalliance.org/lunch-with-docs-pd

## VA Veteran's Centers

- **Focus:** Local support groups and wellness sessions
- **Link:** va.gov *(search "Parkinson's support groups" by location)*

## SPEAK OUT! Home Practice Sessions

- **Focus:** Daily speech therapy sessions
- **Link:** parkinsonvoiceproject.org

## PD Health @ Home

- **Focus:** Virtual wellness and education sessions
- **Link:** parkinson.org/pdhealth

## Getting Support

- **Focus:** Find local support groups
- **Link:** parkinson.org/support (Phone: 1-800-473-4636)

## Facebook Groups

- **Focus:** Explore PD-related support groups
- **Link:** facebook.com *(use "Groups" tab)*

## Faith Communities

- **Focus:** Local congregations may offer caregiver

support
- **Link:** Ask your local church or synagogue

# Part V – Local and Regional Resources

*These resources are specific to certain regions but may inspire you to search for similar services in your own community. Many offer free guides, support groups, and caregiver training.*

### Caregiver Coalition of San Diego

- **Support:** Free handbook, support groups, educational events
- **Website:** caregivercoalitionsd.org

### Parkinson Society British Columbia

- **Support:** Webinars, support groups, caregiver resources
- **Website:** parkinson.bc.ca

### Parkinson Alberta

- **Support:** Local chapters, support groups, educational events
- **Website:** parkinsonassociation.ca

### Parkinson Society Southwestern Ontario

- **Support:** Caregiver guides, support groups, local events
- **Website:** psso.ca

Parkinson Québec

- **Support:** French-language resources, support groups, webinars
- **Website:** parkinsonquebec.ca

# Part V – Intimacy and Connection

*These resources address emotional closeness, communication, and intimacy—important aspects of caregiving that are often overlooked.*

Parkinson's Foundation – Emotional Health

- **Focus:** Mental health, intimacy, and relationships
- **Website:** parkinson.org/emotional-health

Michael J. Fox Foundation – Relationships

- **Focus:** Navigating relationships and communication
- **Website:** michaeljfox.org/relationships

Caregiver.org – Intimacy and Caregiving

- **Focus:** Articles and tips on maintaining intimacy
- **Website:** caregiver.org

- **Focus:** Emotional and spiritual support
- **Website:** Search local congregations or counseling centers

# Part V – Tools and Apps

*These digital tools help with medication tracking, symptom monitoring, and caregiver organization. Many are free or low-cost.*

## Empaira

- **Function:** Community, support, care
- **Platform:** iOS, Android
- **Website:** myempaira.com

## CareZone

- **Function:** Medication tracking, calendar, journal
- **Platform:** iOS, Android
- **Website:** carezone.com

## Medisafe

- **Function:** Pill reminders, drug interaction alerts
- **Platform:** iOS, Android
- **Website:** medisafeapp.com

Parkinson's Tracker App

- **Function:** Symptom tracking and reporting
- **Platform:** iOS, Android
- **Website:** Search app stores for "Parkinson's Tracker"

Google Home / Google Keep / Evernote

- **Function:** Front door camera, reminders, voice assistance, notes, reminders, shared lists
- **Platform:** iOS, Android, Web
- **Websites:** https://home.google.com/welcome https://workspace.google.com/products/keep/

VA Caregiver App Directory

- **Function:** Curated apps for veterans and caregivers
- **Website:** mobile.va.gov/appstore

# Closing Note

*These resources are just a starting point. If you're feeling overwhelmed, remember: you don't have to do this alone. Reach out, explore, and take one step at a time. You are not just a caregiver—you are a lifeline.*

# About the Author

Donna Hauger grew up on a farm near Fergus Falls, Minnesota, where early lessons in resilience and resourcefulness shaped her lifelong love of learning. She earned her B.S. in elementary education from the University of Minnesota, Moorhead, and later completed her master's degree at St. Mary's University of Minnesota.

Her teaching career spanned classrooms from Fertile, Minnesota to Dachau and Augsburg, Germany, and across districts in Spring Lake Park and Rosemount-Eagan, Minnesota. Donna served as a classroom teacher, Reading Recovery specialist, and instructional coach—always with a passion for helping children find their voice through reading and writing. She later taught graduate courses at Hamline University and Capella University, and consulted with school districts nationwide, guiding educators in literacy instruction and student engagement.

Donna's dedication to literacy earned her speaking invitations at the International Reading Association's Conference in Stavanger, Norway, and the Reading Recovery National Conference Banquet in Baltimore, Maryland. Even after retiring in 2016, she continued to volunteer in her West Des Moines neighborhood, supporting young readers and writers.

In 2021, when her husband Daryl was diagnosed with Parkinson's, Donna stepped into a new role: care-partner. From day one, she began journaling—first to cope, then to reflect, and ultimately to connect. Those entries became the foundation for this memoir, a heartfelt offering to fellow caregivers navigating the complexities of love, loss, and adaptation.

Today, Donna and Daryl live in a handicapped-accessible apartment above their son's detached garage—a space filled with grace, grit, and quiet moments of joy. Donna devotes her time to caregiving, writing, and sharing the lessons she's learned with others walking similar paths.

www.ingramcontent.com/pod-product-compliance
Lightning Source LLC
Chambersburg PA
CBHW022332280326
41934CB00006B/611